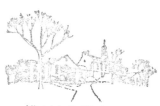

# PACIFIC LIGHT COOKING

ALSO BY RUTH LAW

INDIAN LIGHT COOKING

THE SOUTHEAST ASIA COOKBOOK

DIM SUM—FAST AND FESTIVE CHINESE COOKING

# PACIFIC LIGHT COOKING

## RUTH LAW

### DONALD I. FINE BOOKS
NEW YORK

*To my family,*
*with love*

Donald I. Fine Books
Published by the Penguin Group
Penguin Putnam Inc., 375 Hudson Street, New York, New York 10014, U.S.A.
Penguin Books Ltd, 27 Wrights Lane, London W8 5TZ, England
Penguin Books Australia Ltd, Ringwood, Victoria, Australia
Penguin Books Canada Ltd, 10 Alcorn Avenue, Toronto, Ontario, Canada M4V 3B2
Penguin Books (N.Z.) Ltd, 182–190 Wairau Road, Auckland 10, New Zealand

Penguin Books Ltd, Registered Offices: Harmondsworth, Middlesex, England

First published by Donald I. Fine Books, an imprint of Penguin Putnam Inc.

First Printing, March, 1998
10   9   8   7   6   5   4   3   2   1

LIBRARY OF CONGRESS CATALOGING IN PUBLICATION DATA:
Law, Ruth.
Pacific light cooking / by Ruth Law.
p.   cm.
Includes index.
ISBN 1-556-11519-9
1. Cookery, Oriental.   2. Cookery—Pacific Area.   3. Low-fat diet—Recipes.   I. Title.
TX724.5.A1L34   1998
641.595—dc21                                                97-28630
CIP

Printed in the United States of America
Set in Cochin

BOOKS ARE AVAILABLE AT QUANTITY DISCOUNTS WHEN USED TO PROMOTE
PRODUCTS OR SERVICES. FOR INFORMATION PLEASE WRITE TO
PREMIUM MARKETING DIVISION, PENGUIN PUTNAM INC.,
375 HUDSON STREET, NEW YORK, NEW YORK 10014.

# ACKNOWLEDGMENTS

WHEN I first visited the Pacific Rim eighteen years ago, I was enchanted by the warm hospitality of the people I met, many of whom have become friends. I continue to value my relationship with them and want to thank them and their colleagues who taught me to love their countries.

No book of this kind can be written without a great deal of help in all of its stages. I am deeply obliged to many individuals for their invaluable assistance:

To the many home cooks, chefs, and food experts in both Asia and North America who opened their homes and their kitchens to me and shared their knowledge and lore with me.

To my son Grant and his wife, Mary, who support me in all of my endeavors. Special thanks to Grant for assisting me during my computer dilemmas.

To my many students and tour participants to the Pacific for inspiring me and contributing numerous suggestions and ideas.

Special thanks to Janice Matsumoto for her friendship and constant advice and support, as well as her editing of all things Japanese.

Appreciation to my dedicated agent, Linda Hayes, for her enthusiasm and unwavering attention to detail and for always being there when I need her; to my copy editor, Susan Derecskey, who aided me in untold ways; to Chris Pappas for contributing his artistic talents for the book's illustrations; to Heidi Cusick, who helped me improve my writing skills; to Shirley Corriher, for her valuable food chemistry knowledge; to Howard Deese, Marine Programs Specialist, State of Hawaii, Department of Economic Development and Tourism for his hospitality and for sharing with me his passion for and knowledge of the fishes of Hawaii.

I am extremely grateful to Motoko Abe, wife of Tomoyuki Abe, Consul General of Japan in Chicago who invited me into her kitchen to show me the secrets of Japanese cooking. As author of *Quick & Easy Japanese Cooking*, she helped in checking the Japanese recipes; her eagle eye was much appreciated. I am also indebted to Joelina Soejono, wife of Soejono Soerjoatmodjo, Consul General of Indonesia in Chicago, for showing me her expertise in Indonesian cooking and for reviewing her recipes to assure their accuracy.

I extend my sincere gratitude for advice, counsel, and numerous other contributions to

Edward Robert Brooks Sr., Kathy Carberry, Annette Cremin, Ross Harano, Tad Hillery, Carol McGrath, Bette Peters, Flo and Jack Urhausen, and Cindy Wills.

In addition, I want to thank the executives and staffs of several organizations for coordinating my culinary adventures and helping me with travel arrangements: Hawaii Visitors Bureau, Hong Kong Tourist Association, Consulate General of India, India Tourist Office, Japan National Tourist Organization, Korea National Tourism Corporation, Consulate General of the Republic of Indonesia, Malaysia Tourist Promotion Board, Philippines Department of Tourism, Singapore Tourist Promotion Board, Royal Thai Consulate General, Tourism Authority of Thailand.

And finally, I would like to thank most sincerely all of the many others who assisted me in my latest venture.

# FOREWORD

Y OU'VE HEARD of Murphy's Law? Well, let me tell you about Law's Laws. Law's Laws are more than a set of rules and principles. They're a wonderfully balanced and deeply heartfelt approach to cooking. Now, Ruth Law herself might not actually call them "Law's Laws," but I do. And over the more than fifteen years that I've been a friend and colleague of Ruth's, I've had the pleasure of watching Law's Laws evolve. Here, as I see them, are the principles that make her cooking and writing special.

***The Law of the Source*** — Ruth Law is not one of those food writers whose idea of research is a trip to the library. She knows that if you're going to write about the cuisine of a country, the best way to fire up your imagination and wake up your taste buds is to hop on an airplane. She's done a lot of hopping to and from Asia during the last eighteen years. And we're not just talking about casual sightseeing. When Ruth visits a country, watch out! She'll find her way into the kitchens of chefs and villagers. She'll spend hours wandering through markets, poking, sniffing, gesturing, and tasting — a notebook and camera in one hand and a bag full of exotic ingredients and spices in the other. The mysteries and magic of food are Ruth's passion and her life's work.

***The Law of Lore and Culture*** — Why do people all over the world open their doors and their kitchen cabinets to Ruth Law? It's more than her personality. It's the deep sense of respect and intelligence that she brings. The questions she asks. Her unending fascination with the cooking traditions, the customs, the lore, and, most of all, the people behind the recipes. That's what you'll find in this book: recipes from real cooks — home cooks, chefs at elegant restaurants, enterprising street vendors — who share Ruth's love for authentic foods and flavors.

***The Law of Flavor*** — Now, when Ruth returns to the United States and begins to write up the treasured recipes she brings back from Asia, that's where the real magic begins. Because she has a rare talent for translating Asian cooking methods, tools, and ingredients to make them "user-friendly" for Western cooks without sacrificing flavor. For Ruth, flavor is the bottom line. She's not a stickler for authenticity just for the sake of authenticity, but she knows just what to adapt and what to leave alone to make a dish sizzle and sing. Take one bite of her Grilled Chicken with Balinese Barbecue Sauce and you'll taste what I'm talking about.

*The Law of Simplicity* — I've spent years telling students and TV viewers that much of the food of Asia is remarkably simple to prepare, once you master a few basic techniques. Ruth has always had a deep appreciation for that simplicity. Her recipes are brief and easy to understand — no more and no less than they should be. Coaxing deep, satisfying flavors out of a few basic ingredients is a true art, and Ruth is a master at keeping ingredient lists short and sweet. You won't need to take a laptop computer to the store to remember what to buy. And you won't have to spend all day in the kitchen cooking, either, because the cooking methods are quick and easy to follow. Check out her recipe for "Chilled Tofu." What could be simpler or more perfectly delicious?

*The Law of Light* — Ruth's approach to lighter cooking is a natural one. She begins with the already light and healthful dishes of Asia; then she looks at some of the traditionally heavier Asian fare, and finds ingenious ways to cut down on fat and cholesterol, while still turning out tasty results. That's what sets this book apart from so many other Asian cookbooks: The recipes are consistently designed to be part of a healthful diet. And each one even comes with its own pedigree attached — a nutritional analysis — proving that when it comes to fat and flavor, less really can be more.

You know, people are always asking me for tips and tricks to make cooking lighter. And there are plenty of them, many of which you'll learn just by cooking the recipes in this book. But as Ruth Law knows, lighter cooking is more than just a matter of cutting back and substituting ingredients. It's all about using your instincts and balancing what you eat.

Lighter, more healthful cooking is a way of life that involves eating fresh foods when they're in season, sticking with wholesome ingredients, and giving yourself and the people you love a lively, varied diet that doesn't get bogged down with old-standbys left over from less enlightened times. It's the kind of cooking I grew up on in China — lots of fresh produce and rice, meat used as a condiment rather than a main ingredient, simple sauces designed to enhance the natural flavors of the food.

Which is, after all, what Law's Laws are all about: making small adjustments rather than radical changes; savoring the joy of true flavors; reveling not in rich sauces, but in the richness of culinary traditions. Spend a few minutes with Ruth Law, and suddenly, the challenge of lighter cooking and the mysteries of Asian foods seem a lot less intimidating and a whole lot more fun. Don't you wish all laws were such a pleasure to follow?

— CHEF MARTIN YAN of *Yan Can Cook*

# CONTENTS

# INTRODUCTION

My FASCINATION with the Pacific Rim is boundless. Getting to know the people, their lifestyles, culture, and traditions through a mutual interest in food is a continuing love affair. It began with my first visit when I discovered how central food is to life in the cultures around the Pacific. For over eighteen years, I have traveled through Asia, India, and Hawaii collecting recipes; observing and working with chefs and home cooks; attending cooking schools; eating the foods of street vendors; and talking with people in their kitchens and in the markets. I have come to appreciate the people, who are as subtle and interesting as their cuisines.

Everywhere I've visited food is a topic of conversation, a serious study, a source of daily anticipation. The Chinese on the mainland, as well as in Hong Kong, Taiwan, and Singapore, greet each other not with the familiar how are you? but by asking *chile fan mei you?* (have you had your rice today?).

To most Asians, rice is synonymous with food. Rice is the staple carbohydrate for both the rich and the poor. Meat, vegetables, and fish act as accompaniments to the center of the meal, which is a bowl of rice. It comes in many forms: long grain, extra long grain, short grain, glutinous (or sweet), white, brown, basmati, and jasmine are just a few. It is also ground into a powder to make rice cakes, rice paper, and noodles.

Noodles are a staple in the cooler climates. The Chinese serve noodles for birthday parties and celebrations because they symbolize longevity. In addition to rice, noodles are made from wheat and buckwheat; mung beans ground to a smooth powder for bean threads; and from bean curd pressed into bean noodles. Another staple, gleaming white bean curd, or tofu, acts as a protein-packed foil for spices and sauces.

Along with rice, the common thread among the cuisines is the use of very fresh foods— shimmering just-caught fish, tender farm-raised vegetables, and fruits of the season. In all instances, foods are served at the peak of their season, when they are at their very best. The emphasis is on good taste, aesthetic appearance, and methods of preparation.

While many of the Pacific Rim dishes from Hawaii to India are good for you, some are not. In parts of Southeast Asia, coconut milk, which is high in saturated fat, is a common ingredient. Some Indians use a lot of heavy cream and ghee (clarified butter). And many Asians have a penchant for deep-fried foods. In my recipes, I made substitutes for these ingredients and cooking methods to produce healthy versions with minimal loss of flavor. Using nonstick pans and inspired doses of herbs and spices has the not surprising result of making tastes change. Incorporating these techniques on a daily basis not only lessens the desire for heavy sauces and large pieces of meat but makes eating in a light, healthful manner satisfying.

While different regions of each country have their own emphasis and specialties, they also have ingredients and seasonings in common. Spices native to Southeast Asia and India include cloves, cinnamon, coriander, cardamom, cumin, nutmeg, turmeric, and pepper. Characteristic blends distinguish many dishes. Garlic, ginger, shallots, green onions, fresh coriander (cilantro), soy sauce or fish sauce, and sometimes coconut milk are the ever-present ingredients that merge flavors together. Many dishes are hot with chilies, but they are just part of the spectrum. Sweet, sour, hot, bitter, and salty flavors typically appear in one dish, awakening all of the senses. The importance of balance and variety is found in meals all around the Pacific. This means a fiery dish is served with a mild one, a sweet one with a salty or sour counterpart. Signature dishes from specific regions of each country are attributed to the diversity of terrain, climate, natural resources, and religious beliefs.

Most of the food cooked in these countries is inherently healthful. Steaming and cooking in broths rather than oil is prevalent. One method, done fondue-style at the table, marks special occasions in China, Japan, and Korea. The Mongolian Hot Pot begins with a broth in which thin slices of raw meat, fresh vegetables, tofu, and bean thread noodles are simmered and then served with flavorful sauces. Japan's *Shabu Shabu* and *Yosenabe* are similar dishes. Throughout my travels I searched out the lightest and most interesting dishes. The recipes here are for every day. They are bold, bright, and suitable for company, too.

An overview highlighting the customary cooking methods and popular dishes from countries around the Pacific lends an appetizing introduction to the recipes which follow.

# CHINA

China is the largest country bordering the Pacific. Since the twelfth century, Beijing has been the seat of the government as well as a great cultural and intellectual center. The staggering wealth of the emperors and aristocrats attracted the finest chefs, who brought with them their best dishes from all over the country. Extravagant banquets, sometimes lasting three days, were commonplace. Many of the chefs started restaurants featuring the food from their native regions — Canton, Sichuan, Fukien, Shanghai, Mongolia — making Beijing the culinary capital of northern China.

In the cooler northern climate around Beijing, where rice doesn't grow well, many of the dishes are wheat and soybean based. Steamed breads, dumplings, and wheat flour noodles are flavored with garlic, ginger, green onions, and onions. Potstickers, Mongolian Grilled Ginger Lamb Kabobs, and Mongolian Hot Pot are specialties of this area.

In southern Guangzhou (Canton), the climate is warm and the land fertile. Large rice crops and a wide assortment of vegetables and fruits are grown. Generally, the Cantonese season with soy sauce, rice wine, and ginger and concentrate on enhancing the natural tastes and fragrances of the main ingredients. Stir-fried, roasted, and steamed dishes predominate; Steak Kow in Oyster Sauce and Lemon Chicken are a few specialties. The Cantonese are masters of those filled dumplings and buns known as dim sum. Dim sum means "touch the heart" and these appetizers, traditionally served in teahouses, have stolen mine. I have relished sweet and savory *Shao Mai*, Pearl Balls, and eight-treasure rice packages in lotus leaves in the teahouses of Guangzhou, where as many as sixty varieties of dim sum have been offered to me.

Shanghai, the largest seaport, is the culinary center for the eastern region. The Yangtze River irrigates a profusion of delta-raised fruits and vegetables. The region's style of cooking is dependent on the use of soy sauce balanced with prudent amounts of sugar. Shaohsing produces rice wine, which adds pungency to many dishes. Vinegars from Chekiang are prominent in sweet-and-sour dishes. In the cool winter months, wheat and barley provide grain for the dumplings and noodles. Regional specialties include so-called red-cooked dishes—that is, foods that are simmered in soy sauce until the liquid evaporates, leaving a red hue, and Chinese Five-Treasure Vegetable Platter.

The hot, humid climate of subtropical Sichuan is known for its highly spiced foods. Hot, sour, sweet, and salty flavors are found in many recipes. Sichuan peppercorns, star anise, dried tangerine peel, chilies, garlic, ginger, vinegar, and sugar are vital to the cooking. When in season, oranges, tangerines, and kumquats are enjoyed. Sichuan Stir-fried Orange Beef, Sichuan Noodles with Peanut Sauce, and Sichuan Green Beans are native to this area.

# JAPAN

Japan's culinary approach is characterized by a strong spirit and philosophy. The food exemplifies subtlety of taste, balance of textures, and aesthetic appearance and incorporates serving traditions and settings. Ingredients reflect the four distinct seasons. The placement of equal emphasis on the flavors and textures of each ingredient separates the Japanese style from other Asians, who blend seasonings and main ingredients together to produce an explosion of flavors in your mouth. This meticulous attention to detail, appealing to both the eye and the palate, is an art that ranks Japanese cuisine among the best in the world.

The pinnacle of Japanese cooking is known as *kaiseki-ryori*. It is a highly refined style of cooking which originated with the Buddhist monks who served small snacks called *sado* before the tea ceremony. Located in tranquil garden settings, kaiseki-ryori restaurants elevate the snack to an elaborate refinement meal. Each item is artfully prepared and served on exquisite plates. The plates, often antique porcelain or lacquerware, are chosen to harmonize with the color and texture of the food. Simplicity of the garnish and the seasonal bounty are integral to the meal. No effort is spared to create balance and harmony, including the architecture of the room, the placement of the ikebana flower arrangement, and even the kimonos of the servers. In Kyoto I participated in several of these dinners, which epitomize the highest of Japanese culinary art. Kaiseki-ryori by no means represents Japanese cuisine as a whole, but it plays an important part in understanding the Japanese food philosophy.

The staple foods of Japan are rice, fish, soybean products, seaweed, vegetables, and fruit. The main starch is rice, but udon (wheat noodles) and soba (buckwheat noodles) are also served. Soy sauce, mirin (sweet rice wine), sake (strong rice wine), miso, sesame oil, fresh and pickled ginger are used sparingly to accent the food. Fresh or dried seafood is served at every meal. Dashi, a stock made from kelp and dried bonito flakes, is the base of most soups and many sauces.

# KOREA

Korean food is divided into two distinct types of cooking: the complex, intricately seasoned elegant food of the old courts and the simpler home cooking of the common people. Much time is spent preparing the meal, which, as in other Asian countries, is a major source of enjoyment.

Koreans hold their culinary professionals in high esteem. While in Seoul, I cooked with Chung Hea Han, an acclaimed food authority, cooking school owner, and author of *Korean Cooking*. She is considered a national treasure by the Korean government. She introduced me to the spicy nuances of Korean cuisine, which is seasoned with garlic, ginger, green onions, red pepper powder, sesame oil, soy sauce, and sesame seeds. *Bulgogi* (grilled beef) and *Chap Chae* (a combination of potato starch noodles with vegetables and a little beef or chicken) are classic representatives.

At the onset of winter, Korean housewives prepare a large supply of Kimchi, the national vegetable dish served at every meal. This highly seasoned fermented pickle of cabbage, turnips, cucumber, and other seasonal vegetables provides a good source of vitamins.

# VIETNAM

In Vietnam the food in the north is heavily influenced by the Chinese, who invaded and occupied the region for nearly ten centuries. Their influence is still felt in the many stir-fry dishes and the use of chopsticks. *Nuoc Mam*, fish sauce made from fermented anchovies, imparts a salty flavor, lighter and slightly different from its soy sauce counterpart in China. The Vietnamese penchant for wrapping meats, vegetables, and herbs in lettuce packets is a likely remnant of ancient pre-Chinese civilizations.

France and India influenced the foods of southern Vietnam. Dishes are customarily spicier, sweeter, and heartier than those in the north. Cooked foods are often combined with crisp raw vegetables and aromatic herbs such as mint, fresh coriander, and basil. Tropical fruits, sugarcane, chilies, a plethora of vegetables, coconut trees, and rice crops abound in the fertile fields around the Mekong River. Coconut milk is a common ingredient, as are chilies, pineapples, tomatoes, and bean sprouts. Here you'll find classic Southeast Asian fare such as stir-fries as well as long loaves of crusty baguettes and pâtés, reminders of the French influence.

Rice is the main dish throughout Vietnam. Variations of *Nuoc Cham*, a refreshing yet hot sauce made from fish sauce, lime, garlic, chilies, and sugar, are found on the table at most meals. Nuoc Cham is used as a dipping sauce and to season the food.

# THAILAND

Thailand has been called "the land of a thousand smiles." The first smile comes from dining on Thai food, which invariably leaves a pleasant aftertaste that lingers long after the meal is finished. Every dish induces, in me at least, another smile. I can't wait for the next bite.

Contrasting ingredients signify *Pad Thai* (a noodle and shrimp combination) and Spicy Thai Chicken Salad, a northern favorite. Although many dishes are quite fiery, chilies are only a part of the synchronized blending of flavors. Other typical seasonings include garlic, ginger, galangal, lemon grass, fresh coriander, shallots, mint, a blend of spices — peppercorns, cloves, nutmeg, cardamom, cinnamon, cumin — and a touch of nam pla, fish sauce made from salted and fermented anchovies similar to the Vietnamese nuoc mam.

An aromatic, fiery, and tantalizingly seasoned Thai meal isn't considered complete without soup and plenty of rice. Soup is devoured from dawn to dusk. Frequently it is served on top of the rice. Thai fruits, with their spectacular tastes, shapes, and colors, add a refreshing dimension. Many are artfully carved into elaborate flowers and leaves to enhance the table centerpiece or plate presentation.

# SINGAPORE

You might expect that Singapore's food would reflect its Chinese heritage. For the most part, the cuisine of this small island of 224 square miles — the size of the city of Chicago and only a fifth the size of the state of Rhode Island—is a cultural melting pot of Chinese, Malay, and Indian inhabitants. The food has great diversity as well as a harmonious exchange of cooking ingredients and techniques contributed by these and other resident ethnic groups.

My favorite is also one of the most distinctive styles—*nonya*, or Straits Chinese cuisine, created when Chinese male immigrants to the Straits settlements of Singapore, Penang, and Malacca took Malay wives. Their descendants are known either as Peranaken or Straits Chinese. The wives are called nonyas and the men *babas*. Nonya food is that served in the home of a nonya woman. Chinese implements and methods and local ingredients, such as coconut milk, turmeric, ginger, galangal, shallots, chives, candlenuts, shrimp paste, lemon grass, limes, tamarind, green mangoes, and a wealth of chilies produce the nonya blend of robust and spicy cooking. A classic example is Beef Rendang, which is a fiery curry. Nonya desserts are extremely sweet.

# THE PHILIPPINES

The Philippines, an archipelago of 7,107 islands lying between the Pacific Ocean and the China Sea, is an intersection of many cultures—Malay, Chinese, Spanish, Hindu, Muslim, and American. The strongest influences come from the Chinese with their rice and noodle dishes and the Spanish with their sautéed and stewed dishes.

Although the Spanish influence is felt mostly in the cooking of the elite, the accent is indelible all over the islands. They brought olive oil to use in place of coconut oil and hearty stews like *calderetta*, made from beef or goat. They introduced afternoon tea and fiesta fare, including the pit-cooking of *lechon*, a large pig grilled over coals.

The Filipinos have changed and adapted the foods of their immigrants using local ingredients. The wealth of seafood around the islands and the tropical climate encourage the abundant use of fruits, coconuts, and tamarind. As in other parts of Asia, ginger, garlic, and onions are primary flavorings. The proximity to Southeast Asia is noticeable by the use of fermented shrimp paste, *bagoong*, and fish sauce, *patis*. Quite an array of small portions of dipping sauces called *sawsawan* are important condiments. Sauces containing vinegar with crushed garlic go with pork dishes and chicken *adobo*, and *bagoong* with lime juice accompanies grilled fish. There's always a bottle of vinegar and red chilies on the table to be added as desired.

# INDONESIA

Indonesia encompasses thirteen thousand islands, stretching a distance of 3,200 miles from Sumatra in the west to the coast of Irian Jaya in the east. With flavors to rival any of the world's cuisines, the cooking blends the influences of different ethnic and religious groups, of which Muslim is predominant everywhere except Bali, which is Hindu. Once known as the Spice Islands, Indonesia was a major trading crossroads and incorporated the culinary preferences of the Middle East, Portugal, the Netherlands, China, and India with its own native dishes.

With Indonesian food, your tastebuds can expect a great awakening. Although known for heat, every Indonesian dish is not fiery. Marvelous combinations of textures and colors are integrated with sweet, sour, spicy, bitter, and salty flavors. For each spicy dish, a cooling one balances it; for each sweet one, a salty or sour dish is served.

As elsewhere in Asia, rice is central to every meal. Unlike the Chinese and Japanese, the Indonesians mix rice with other cooked foods. They serve the mixtures with fiery sambals, prepared from chilies and spices. Red and green chili sambals are omnipresent table condiments, which are used for spicing each dish to taste.

Indonesian foods vary from island to island. Satay, grilled meat on a skewer, however, could be called a national dish. It seems that every chef in every town has a personal variation of the satay peanut sauce and a special technique for marinating the meat before grilling. Throughout the country dishes with the same name might be made of different ingredients. In my travels I heard lengthy discussions about the correct method of preparing and seasoning a particular dish. In this book, I used ingredients and cooking methods from the place where I first learned the dish.

One method found throughout the islands is the wrapping of food in a fragrant banana leaf or palm frond and then steaming or grilling it. An example is Balinese Grilled Sea Bass in a Banana Leaf. (I have substituted sea bass for the local fish.) Everywhere fresh fish is combined with such vegetables as green beans, cabbage, cucumber, eggplant, tomatoes, and bean sprouts. These are cooked together or tossed into salads, like *Gado Gado*, and seasoned with shallots, ginger, garlic, turmeric, chilies, fresh coriander, tamarind, sugar, and *kecap manis*, a sweet soy sauce. Indigenous fruits like mangosteen, with its smooth deep purple shell and five pearly white, sweet-sour segments, are served as superlative desserts.

# MALAYSIA

Malaysia shares similar cooking traditions with Indonesia. Many of the people of both countries have Malay roots. In addition to the Malays, the Malaysian population is 32 percent Chinese and ten percent Indian. All of this is reflected in the cuisine. Coming from one of the world's largest exporters, pepper is a major seasoning. The curries of the Malay rely heavily on lemon grass, galangal, chilies, citrus, fresh coriander, and curry leaves. Coconut is the basis of the curries as well as many other dishes. Traditional Chinese dishes such as spring rolls are spiced with cinnamon. And fare from Borneo, such as pickled mackerel and hot and sour oxtail soup, finds its way into the cuisine.

# INDIA

Diversity best describes the cooking of India. There, as everywhere, geography, history, cultural heritage, and religious beliefs contribute to the way food is prepared. This subcontinent of well over a million square miles is divided into twenty-five states, each with its own language, dress, customs, and cooking style. Not only that, but each style of cooking has many different schools, with each school having more than one style. In my book *Indian Light Cooking*, I cover the kitchens of India in detail. Generally speaking, it can be said that Indian cooking can be broadly viewed as having two main culinary divisions. The food of the north is predominantly wheat based; the food of the south, rice based.

Most of India's population are Hindus; they do not consume beef because the cow is considered sacred. The Hindu Brahmins of Bengal eat a lot of fish and shellfish. The southern Hindus, who are mainly vegetarians, have created highly spiced, colorful dishes, sometimes sauced with coconut milk. The Moghuls of the north, with their Central Asian Muslim cuisine, have devised melt-in-your-mouth lamb and mutton combinations and elaborate meat and rice pilafs known as *biryanis*.

The process of baking, roasting, and grilling in the *tandoor*, a coal-fueled clay pit, is thought to have originated in Persia. Baked flat breads or *nans*, *Murgh Tikka* (spiced chicken kabobs), and the well-known tandoori chicken are specialties of the tandoor.

In the tropical coastal area of Goa, formerly a Portuguese state, the population is predominately Catholic. The Portuguese, once the world's spice traders, brought spices and chilies to produce fiery hot and spicy lamb, pork, beef, and fish curries known as *vindaloos*. There are other minorities in India such as the Parsis on the west coast who fled Muslim persecution in Persia in the eighth century, the Syrian Christians of Kerala, and the reformed Hindu community of Jains—each with its own unique cooking style. No wonder it is hard to define Indian cuisine!

The heart of Indian cuisine everywhere is *masala*, a fragrant blend of herbs and spices which make each dish distinctive. Masalas can be wet or dry. Wet masalas are ground daily. The pastes contain chilies, ginger, garlic, onion, lime juice or tamarind, nutmeg, cinnamon, cardamom, cloves, cumin, fennel, coriander, and turmeric in proportions personalized to each dish by the cook. Dry masalas, such as Garam Masala, contain blends of freshly ground black cardamom seeds, cinnamon, cloves, black peppercorns, and often cumin seeds. Garam Masala is usually sprinkled over a dish before serving or added to the dish at the end of cooking. The possibilities of spice blends are infinite, as each cook employs those of the region to individual tastes. The goal is to produce a perfect spice blend without any one particular spice or flavor predominating.

No Indian meal is complete without one or two *dals* such as Indian Spiced Mung Beans with Spinach and Sweet and Spicy Lentils made from lentils, peas, and beans which are important sources of protein, have no cholesterol, and only a trace of fat. They are also high in carbohydrates, fiber, vitamin B, and minerals. These legumes are combined with vegetables in intriguingly spiced combinations and always consumed with rice or an Indian bread. Side dishes such as chutneys and pickles are important as condiments to balance flavors. Another commonality in Indian cooking is the importance given to flavor, texture, spice, and balance.

# HAWAII

A cookbook about the Pacific without the vibrant foods and fish of Hawaii wouldn't be complete. From this veritable melting pot, a tremendous Asian influence is coupled with Hawaiian-raised produce to create a naturally flavor-intensive cuisine and a harmonious addition to the light fare included here. The Chinese, Filipino, Thai, and Japanese cooking styles redefine the uses of big flavors by using delicate salsas and relishes to serve with simply prepared seafood such as Grilled Mahimahi with Papaya and Maui Onion Relish and Broiled Tuna with Mango Relish. Traditional potstickers and rice and noodle dishes are found, but seem to take on a brighter intensity, perhaps from the close proximity of the sea and sun around these beautiful islands in the middle of the Pacific. Salads such as Chicken Salad with Papaya Seed and Orange-Ginger Dressing and Hawaiian Tropical Salsa provide color.

Hawaii doesn't corner the travelogue on beauty. The Asian countries featured in this book are as beautiful as their food is delicious. Attention to harmony and balance extends from growing the food to cooking it. Sampling these dishes is like taking a mini-trip, and a healthful one. Once the ginger hits the sauté pan, the garlic is stir-fried, the chilies minced, and the fish sauce measured an aromatic journey begins. It continues with preparing vegetables, fruit, grains, and fish, becomes scenic on the plate, and lingers memorably on the palate. This is why I love the cuisines around the Pacific.

# ABOUT THE NUTRITIONAL ANALYSIS OF RECIPES

THE RECIPES in this book were analyzed by Linda R. Yoakam, M.S., R.D., L.D. The information is derived from calculation based on Nutritionist IV, Version 3.5, N-Square Computing, First Data Bank Division, The Hearst Corporation, and the following: *Bowes and Church's Food Values of Portions Commonly Used*, sixteenth edition (J.P. Lippincott Company, Philadelphia, 1994); *The Complete Book of Food Counts*, Corinne T. Netzer (Dell Publishing, New York, 1994); and *Composition of Foods, Agriculture Handbook No. 8* (U.S. Department of Agriculture). *No warranty as to the accuracy of these results is expressed or implied.*

The following applies to the nutritional analysis of recipes.

- When an ingredient is listed as optional, it is not included in the analysis.
- Ingredients added "to taste" are not included in the analysis.
- Suggested accompaniments are not included, unless specific amounts are given.
- The data given is for one serving or unit (such as a dumpling) unless the yield is expressed in cups, when the size of the serving is indicated.
- When a recipe yield is given in a range of serving sizes, the larger number is used. If there is a range in the amount of an ingredient, the smaller amount is used.
- Salt is figured only if a recipe calls for a specific amount.

# STARTERS

SPICED WONTON CRISPS

THAI CORN CAKES WITH PLUM DIPPING SAUCE

INDONESIAN CORN AND SHRIMP FRITTERS (*Pergedel Jagung Udang*)

POTSTICKERS

OPEN-FACED CHICKEN AND SHRIMP DUMPLINGS (*Shao Mai*)

CHINESE PEARL BALLS

SHRIMP, EGGPLANT, AND CARROT SUMMER ROLLS WITH VIETNAMESE DIPPING SAUCE

FILIPINO SHRIMP, TURKEY, AND VEGETABLES IN LETTUCE PACKAGES (**Fresh** *Lumpia*)

KOREAN MIXED VEGETABLES AND CHICKEN LETTUCE PACKAGES WITH MUSTARD
  DIPPING SAUCE (*Gyeoja Char*)

SPICY THAI CHICKEN SALAD (*Larb*)

INDIAN ROASTED EGGPLANT AND TOMATO PUREE (*Baigan Bharta*)

INDIAN SPICED CHICKEN KABOBS WITH MINT-CORIANDER CHUTNEY (*Murgh Tikka*)

CHILLED TOFU (*Hiya-Yakko*)

HAND-WRAPPED SUSHI (*Nigiri-Zushi*)

VINEGARED RICE FOR SUSHI

EASY INDIAN SPICED CHICKEN KABOBS

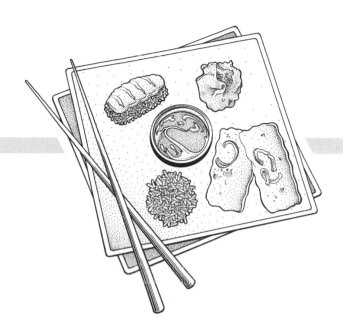

# STARTERS

ASIANS LOVE to snack—before meals, during meals, and after meals. The mouth-watering starters you will find in this chapter are a sampling of the many tidbits found in street stalls, homes, restaurants, and dim sum shops from Shanghai to Honolulu.

When served in your home, they translate to exotic palate teasers. I like to serve a selection of textures and flavors, and not all from just one region. For example, I might set an appetizer buffet with Chinese Pearl Balls and open-faced dumplings, Thai Corn Cakes, and Indian Spiced Chicken Kabobs with an assortment of dipping sauces, such as Mint-Coriander Chutney (page 38 or 237) and Plum Dipping Sauce.

I sometimes treat my guests to a "wrap and roll" party. Using lettuce leaves for the wrap, I set out Filipino Shrimp, Turkey, and Vegetables; Korean Mixed Vegetables and Chicken; Spicy Thai Chicken Salad; and Vietnamese Grilled Beef (page 114). If you cool it all with a refreshing salad like Carrot and Cabbage Slaw (page 213), you may want to skip the entree.

# SPICED WONTON CRISPS

SEASONED WITH ginger, garlic, fresh coriander, and red pepper powder, spiced wontons are a unique alternative to potato chips. They are tasty served alone or with a dip. For a fusion cuisine variation, sprinkle two tablespoons freshly grated parmesan cheese on the wontons instead of the fresh coriander mixture at the end of the baking time. Or for a sweet rendition, sprinkle the cooked crisps with powdered sugar immediately after removing them from the oven.

Wonton crisps will keep, stored in an airtight container, for a month.

> 1/4 pound wonton wrappers (about 18 wrappers)
> Canola oil spray
> 1 tablespoon plus 1 teaspoon coarsely chopped fresh coriander (cilantro)
> 1 clove garlic, coarsely chopped
> 1 1/2 teaspoons peeled and coarsely chopped ginger
> 1/4 to 1/2 teaspoon red pepper powder
> Kosher salt, to taste

Preheat the oven to 375 degrees.

Bring 2 quarts of water to a boil in a large saucepan. Drop half of the wrappers, one at a time, into the boiling water. Cook for 1 to 2 minutes, or until soft but not mushy. Remove and place in a bowl of ice water. Repeat with the remaining wrappers.

Lightly spray 2 large nonstick baking sheets with the oil. Unfold the wonton wrappers individually under water. Remove from the water and arrange them on a cookie sheet in a single layer. Spray the surface of the wontons lightly with the oil. Bake for about 5 minutes, or until they start to brown.

Meanwhile, chop together the fresh coriander, garlic, and ginger until very fine. Stir in the red pepper powder and mix well. Sprinkle a little of the mixture over each of the wontons and continue to bake for 2 to 3 minutes, or until dry and brown. Sprinkle with salt to taste. Serve immediately.

*Yield: 18 crisps*

| | | | |
|---|---|---|---|
| Calories | 19 | Cholesterol | 0 mg |
| Fat | 0 g | Sodium | 36 mg |
| Saturated Fat | 0 g | Carbohydrate | 4 g |
| Mono | 0 g | Protein | 1 g |
| Poly | 0 g | | |

# THAI CORN CAKES WITH PLUM DIPPING SAUCE

THE THAIS love to snack all day! These spiced corn cakes, sold by street vendors, are a favorite. They make a tasty appetizer when accompanied by refreshing Plum Dipping Sauce and/or Hot-and-Sour Cucumbers (page 218). For crisper cakes, deep-fry them in oil as they do in Thailand.

Defrosted frozen corn may be substituted for fresh corn. It is not necessary to blanch frozen corn. The cakes may be cooked ahead and reheated in the oven.

1¾ cups fresh corn kernels (about 4 ears)
½ cup all-purpose flour
½ teaspoon baking powder
¼ teaspoon baking soda
1 teaspoon sugar
Salt, to taste
½ teaspoon freshly ground black pepper
½ to 1 teaspoon red pepper powder
¾ cup buttermilk
2 teaspoons canola oil
1 tablespoon finely chopped fresh coriander (cilantro) leaves
3 teaspoons minced garlic
3 tablespoons minced shallot
1 to 2 teaspoons fish sauce
Canola oil spray

*Plum Dipping Sauce*
½ cup plum sauce
2 tablespoons dry sherry
¼ teaspoon ground cinnamon

Blanch the corn until crisp-tender. Sift the flour, baking powder, baking soda, sugar, salt, black pepper, and red pepper powder together in a bowl. Combine the buttermilk and oil and add to the dry ingredients. Stir just until the dry ingredients are moistened. Stir in the fresh coriander, garlic, shallot, fish sauce, and corn. Mix thoroughly until a thick, lumpy batter is formed.

Combine the plum sauce, sherry, and cinnamon in a small bowl and stir to mix. Set aside.

Heat a large nonstick skillet over medium heat. Lightly spray the pan with oil. Drop heaping tablespoonfuls of the batter onto the pan, spreading each into a 2-inch round. Cook on each side for 2½ to 3 minutes, or until golden. Repeat with the remaining mixture. Serve with the plum dipping sauce.

*Yield: about 16 cakes*

| | | | |
|---|---|---|---|
| Calories | 56 | Cholesterol | 0 mg |
| Fat | 1 g | Sodium | 59 mg |
| Saturated Fat | 0 g | Carbohydrate | 11 g |
| Mono | 0 g | Protein | 2 g |
| Poly | 0 g | | |

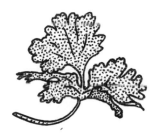

# INDONESIAN CORN
# AND SHRIMP FRITTERS

## PERGEDEL JAGUNG UDANG

THIS DELICATELY spiced corn and shrimp fritter comes from the kitchen of Joelina Soejono, wife of Soejono Soerjoatmodjo, Consul General of Indonesia in Chicago. In Indonesia, she says, the fritters are made from freshly grated sweet corn on the cob. Defrosted frozen corn can be used instead. When preparing the *pergedel*, Joelina uses a combination of green onion and celery leaves, but for ease of preparation, I have used only the green onion. She also deep-fries fritters, but I panfry them in a little oil. In Indonesia, the fritters are served as a snack or as an accompaniment to a meal.

The pergedel can be made ahead and frozen. Reheat in a 350 degree oven.

> 1³/₄ cups frozen corn, defrosted
> 4 ounces shrimp, minced
> 2 cloves garlic, minced
> 3 shallots, minced
> 1 green onion, minced
> 2 eggs, lightly beaten
> ¹/₄ cup all-purpose flour
> ¹/₃ teaspoon white pepper
> Sugar, to taste
> Salt, to taste
> 1 to 2 teaspoons canola oil
> Canola oil spray (optional)

In a large bowl, crush the corn slightly with a wooden spoon. Stir in the shrimp, garlic, shallots, and green onion. Add the eggs and stir. Add the flour and stir to combine. The mixture should be slightly moist. Add the white pepper and season with sugar and salt. Stir to combine thoroughly.

Heat a large nonstick skillet over medium heat. Add 1 teaspoon oil. Drop a heaping tablespoonful of the batter onto the pan. Cook on each side for 2¹/₂ to 3 minutes per side, or until golden and cooked through. Repeat with the remaining mixture, adding more oil if necessary. If desired, lightly spray the cooked fritters with a touch of canola oil. Serve hot.

*Yield: about 20 fritters*

| Calories | 36 | Cholesterol | 30 mg |
|---|---|---|---|
| Fat | 1 g | Sodium | 18 mg |
| Saturated Fat | 0 g | Carbohydrate | 5 g |
| Mono | 0 g | Protein | 2 g |
| Poly | 0 g | | |

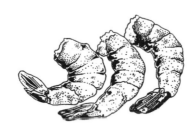

# POTSTICKERS

WHEN IN Beijing, I always stop at a curbside stand to sample these popular dumplings. They have a dual texture through the combined processes of shallow-frying and steaming, making them soft on the top and crisp on the bottom.

If round potsticker or *gyoza* wrappers are unavailable, buy wonton wrappers and cut them into circles with scissors or a round biscuit cutter. The dumplings can be prepared ahead and frozen. Cook just before serving. The dumplings are offered with a variety of sauces; one of the most common is Soy-Vinegar-Sesame Dipping Sauce (page 241).

### Filling
1/2 pound lean ground chicken or pork
1 cup finely chopped Chinese or napa cabbage
3 green onions, minced
4 to 6 Chinese dried black mushrooms, soaked in hot water for 20 minutes,
    stems removed, caps minced
4 teaspoons peeled and minced ginger
1 tablespoon low-sodium soy sauce
1 tablespoon dry sherry
2 teaspoons cornstarch
1/2 teaspoon sugar
1/2 teaspoon salt (optional)
Dash of white pepper

24 potsticker or *gyoza* wrappers
1 1/2 tablespoons canola oil
2/3 cup fat-free low-sodium Chicken Stock (page 60) or water
Dipping sauce

Combine the filling ingredients in a bowl and mix well.

Place a heaping teaspoon of the filling in the center of each wrapper. Brush the outer edges of each wrapper with a little water. Fold the circle in half, forming a half-moon. Starting at one end, with your forefinger and thumb, make 2 to 3 pleats on the back side. Then pinch them together with the front side of the dough to seal the filling. Do the same at the other end until the opening is completely closed. Pinch the edges to seal tightly to prevent the filling from leaking during cooking. Tap the finished dumpling on a flat surface to make a flat bottom. Repeat with the remaining wrappers and filling. When preparing, keep the wrappers and the finished dumplings covered with a towel to prevent drying.

Heat a large heavy nonstick skillet over medium heat. Add half of the oil and swirl around the pan. Arrange half of the dumplings in the pan, seam side up. Cook until the bottoms are golden brown, about 3 to 4 minutes. Add half of the stock to the skillet. Reduce the heat to low. Cover and cook until the liquid is absorbed, 5 to 6 minutes. Remove the dumplings from the pan. Keep warm in a low oven while you repeat the procedure with the remaining dumplings

Place the dumplings, brown side up, on a serving platter. Serve with a dipping sauce on the side.

*Yield: 24 dumplings*

| | | | |
|---|---|---|---|
| Calories | 33 | Cholesterol | 6 mg |
| Fat | 1 g | Sodium | 63 mg |
| Saturated Fat | 0 g | Carbohydrate | 3 g |
| Mono | 1 g | Protein | 3 g |
| Poly | 0 g | | |

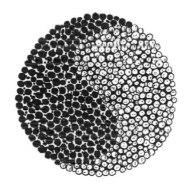

# OPEN-FACED CHICKEN AND SHRIMP DUMPLINGS

## SHAO MAI

IN CHINA, these succulent dumplings are a favorite in the dim sum shops or teahouses. They are usually stuffed with pork, but I prefer this lighter version made with chicken and shrimp. The dumplings make tasty hors d'oeuvres served with Soy-Vinegar-Sesame Dipping Sauce (page 243).

The dumplings can be frozen for one month.

Canola oil spray

### Filling
8 ounces ground chicken breast
8 ounces shrimp, shelled, deveined, and coarsely chopped
6 water chestnuts, coarsely chopped
4 Chinese dried black mushrooms, soaked in hot water for 20 minutes, stems removed, caps coarsely chopped
3 tablespoons chopped green onion
1 tablespoon peeled and chopped fresh ginger
1 teaspoon low-sodium soy sauce
1 teaspoon Asian sesame oil
1 teaspoon dry sherry
$1/2$ teaspoon sugar
Salt and freshly ground black pepper, to taste
$11/2$ teaspoons cornstarch

32 potsticker or *gyoza* or wonton wrappers cut in circles
32 frozen peas, for garnish (optional)
Dipping sauce

Line 2 steamer trays with wax or parchment paper lightly sprayed with the oil or use aluminum pie plates punched with holes and lightly sprayed with oil.

Combine the filling ingredients and mix well to blend evenly.

Place 1 heaping tablespoon of the filling in the center of each wrapper. Gather the edges around the filling to form pleats. Lightly squeeze the center of the dumpling. With a spoon, smooth the meat surface. If desired, lightly press a pea in the center of the filling. Tap the dumpling on a flat surface to make the bottom flat. Cover with a towel while preparing the remaining dumplings.

Arrange the dumplings upright ¹/₂ inch apart on the steamer trays. Fill a wok or large pot with 2 inches of water for steaming and bring to a boil. Stack the steamer trays (or place 1 pie plate of dumplings on a stand) over the boiling water, cover, and steam over high heat for 5 minutes, or until cooked through. Serve the dumplings hot with dipping sauce.

*Yield: 32 dumplings*

| | | | |
|---|---|---|---|
| Calories | 29 | Cholesterol | 15 mg |
| Fat | 0 g | Sodium | 39 mg |
| Saturated Fat | 0 g | Carbohydrate | 3 g |
| Mono | 0 g | Protein | 3 g |
| Poly | 0 g | | |

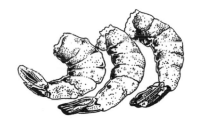

# CHINESE PEARL BALLS

THESE GLISTENING rice dumplings seem to be coated with little pearls. In China, they are stuffed with fish, meat, or chicken. I find turkey, which is readily available in supermarkets, makes a tasty dumpling when combined with traditional flavors. Serve them with Spicy Coriander-Mint Dipping Sauce (page 241) or Soy-Vinegar-Sesame Dipping Sauce (page 243).

Cooked pearl balls can be reheated by steaming over boiling water until warmed through, six to eight minutes.

1$^1$/$_3$ cups glutinous rice
$^3$/$_4$ cup water chestnuts
Canola oil spray
1 pound lean ground turkey
8 Chinese dried black mushrooms, soaked in hot water for 20 minutes, stems removed, caps minced
1$^1$/$_2$ tablespoons peeled and minced fresh ginger
1 tablespoon minced green onion
3 tablespoons low-sodium soy sauce
1 tablespoon dry sherry
1 teaspoon Asian sesame oil
2 tablespoons cornstarch
Dipping sauce

Wash and drain the rice several times until the water runs clear. Drain and transfer to a baking sheet. Set aside.

Blanch the water chestnuts in boiling water for 10 seconds. Drain. Refresh with cold water, drain. Coarsely chop.

Line 1 or 2 steamer trays with wax or parchment paper (or use aluminum pie plates punched with holes) and spray with the oil.

Combine the turkey, mushrooms, water chestnuts, ginger, green onion, soy sauce, sherry, sesame oil, and cornstarch in a bowl and stir to combine thoroughly. Shape the turkey mixture into balls about 1 inch in diameter. Roll each ball in the glutinous rice until well coated with grains, lightly pressing the rice into the ball so it clings.

Arrange the balls on the steamer tray leaving a $^1$/$_2$-inch space between them. Fill a wok or large pot with water for steaming and bring to a boil. Stack the steamer trays over the boiling water or place 1 pie plate of dumplings on a stand over the boiling water. Cover and steam over high heat for 10 minutes, or until the rice and turkey are cooked.

Serve hot drizzled with dipping sauce.

*Yield: about 24 pearl balls*

| | | | |
|---|---|---|---|
| Calories | 67 | Cholesterol | 7 mg |
| Fat | 1 g | Sodium | 74 mg |
| Saturated Fat | 0 g | Carbohydrate | 10 g |
| Mono | 0 g | Protein | 4 g |
| Poly | 0 g | | |

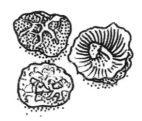

# SHRIMP, EGGPLANT, AND CARROT SUMMER ROLLS WITH VIETNAMESE DIPPING SAUCE

SHRIMP, SPICED eggplant, and carrots topped with sprigs of fresh coriander and mint are wrapped in Vietnamese rice paper, then dipped into a tangy hot sauce. These summer rolls are a perfect appetizer, light luncheon dish, or picnic food.

The rolls may be prepared several hours in advance, covered with plastic wrap, and refrigerated. If the rolls become dry, spray them with warm water, using an atomizer.

### *Vietnamese Dipping Sauce*
4 tablespoons rice vinegar
6 tablespoons fresh lime juice
4 teaspoons fish sauce
1 to 2 red chilies, seeded and minced, or $1/2$ to 1 teaspoon red pepper flakes
2 tablespoons sugar

1 teaspoon canola oil
2 teaspoons peeled and minced fresh ginger
2 cloves garlic, minced
2 shallots, minced
2 medium Japanese eggplants, cut into julienne
10 dried rice paper wrappers, $6^1/2$ inches in diameter
10 Boston lettuce leaves
2 carrots, cut into julienne
1 pound medium shrimp, cooked, shelled, deveined, and cut lengthwise in half
10 sprigs of fresh coriander (cilantro)
10 sprigs fresh mint

Combine the rice vinegar, lime juice, fish sauce, red chili, and sugar in a bowl. Stir to mix. Cover. Refrigerate for at least 20 minutes, stirring occasionally to dissolve the sugar.

Heat the oil in a nonstick skillet over medium heat. Add the ginger, garlic, and shallots. Stir for 20 seconds. Add the eggplant and sauté until soft and tender. Remove from the pan and let cool.

Dip each rice paper wrapper into warm water and place on a flat surface. Allow the paper to soften for 2 to 3 minutes, or until soft and pliable. Alternate dipping the papers and filling the rolls so you will not have to wait for the rice papers to soften. (You may also moisten the rice papers with a pastry brush or spray with an atomizer bottle filled with warm water instead of dipping them in water. Allow to soften before using.)

Center 1 lettuce leaf along the lower third of the rice paper wrapper. Place about 1 1/2 tablespoons of the eggplant mixture, some carrots, and about 3 shrimp pieces on top of the lettuce leaf. Place a sprig of coriander and of fresh mint on the top. Fold in the sides in an envelope pattern and roll up tightly into a 3-inch-long cylinder. Repeat with remaining wrappers. Store in the refrigerator, seam side down. Serve with the dipping sauce.

*Yield: 10 rolls*

| Calories | 387 | Cholesterol | 178 mg |
|---|---|---|---|
| Fat | 4 g | Sodium | 942 mg |
| Saturated Fat | 1 g | Carbohydrate | 61 g |
| Mono | 2 g | Protein | 28 g |
| Poly | 1 g | | |

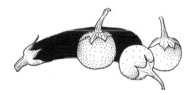

# FILIPINO SHRIMP, TURKEY, AND VEGETABLES IN LETTUCE PACKAGES

### FRESH *LUMPIA*

*LUMPIA,* THE Filipino version of the Chinese egg roll, can be fried or fresh as in this dish. Norma Manankil, a caterer in Westmont, Illinois, who is of Filipino origin, combines shrimp, ground turkey, and crisp vegetables and wraps them in a lettuce leaf. She says you can also wrap the lumpia in rice paper. If desired, serve the rolls with garlic sauce.

**Garlic Sauce (optional)**
1 cup fat-free low-sodium Chicken Stock (page 60)
2 tablespoons sugar
1 teaspoon low-sodium soy sauce
Salt and freshly ground black pepper, to taste
1 tablespoon cornstarch dissolved in 2 tablespoons water
2 cloves garlic, minced

2 teaspoons canola oil
2 cloves garlic, minced
3/4 cup coarsely chopped onion
10 medium shrimp, shelled, deveined, and minced
1/2 pound lean ground turkey or pork
12 fresh green beans, trimmed and cut on the diagonal into 1/4-inch pieces
1 carrot, cut into 1 1/2-inch-long julienne
1/2 cup julienned peeled potatoes
3/4 cup shredded cabbage
3/4 cup fresh bean sprouts
2 tablespoons low-sodium soy sauce
Salt and freshly ground black pepper, to taste
12 romaine or Boston lettuce leaves
1/4 cup chopped peanuts (optional)

To prepare the sauce, combine the stock, sugar, soy sauce, salt, and pepper in a small pan. Cook until the sugar is dissolved. Recombine the cornstarch and add to the pan. Cook, stirring, over medium heat until the sauce thickens and is glossy. Serve the sauce hot, sprinkled with minced garlic.

Heat the oil in a nonstick sauté pan. Add the garlic and onion and stir until translucent, about 2 to 3 minutes. Add the shrimp and turkey and stir-fry for 1 minute. Add the following vegetables a handful at a time: green beans, carrot, potato, cabbage, and bean sprouts. Stir-fry for 2 to 3 minutes, or until the vegetables are tender but still crunchy. Stir in the soy sauce, salt, and pepper. Arrange lettuce leaves around a large platter. Place the filling in the center. If using, sprinkle peanuts over the filling. To eat, put about 2 tablespoons of the filling on a lettuce leaf. Roll up the leaf, turning in the sides so that the filling is enclosed. Serve with warm garlic sauce, if desired.

*Yield: 12 rolls*

| | | | |
|---|---|---|---|
| Calories | 53 | Cholesterol | 16 mg |
| Fat | 1 g | Sodium | 110 mg |
| Saturated Fat | 1 g | Carbohydrate | 5 g |
| Mono | 1 g | Protein | 5 g |
| Poly | 0 g | | |

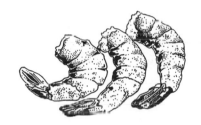

# KOREAN MIXED VEGETABLES AND CHICKEN LETTUCE PACKAGES WITH MUSTARD DIPPING SAUCE

## GYEOJA CHAR

COLORFUL VEGETABLES and chicken are wrapped in a lettuce leaf, then dipped into a sharp mustard sauce in this attractive appetizer taught to me by Chung Hea Han, a Seoul cooking-school owner and author of *Korean Cooking*. She used six ounces of ham cut into matchstick strips but said you could use chicken instead.

1 Bosc pear, peeled, cored, and cut into 1½-inch-long julienne
2 teaspoons fresh lemon juice
1 egg, lightly beaten (optional)

### Mustard Dipping Sauce
¼ cup boiling water
1 to 2 tablespoons hot mustard powder
2 teaspoons sesame seeds, toasted
2 tablespoons rice vinegar
2 tablespoons sugar
2 tablespoons low-sodium soy sauce
2 teaspoons Asian sesame oil

5 water chestnuts, sliced
6 romaine lettuce leaves
6 ounces cooked boneless and skinless chicken breasts, cut into 1½-inch-long julienne
1 medium cucumber, seeded and cut into 1½-inch-long julienne
1 small carrot, cut into 1½-inch-long julienne

Combine the pear, lemon juice, and water to cover in a bowl to prevent darkening. Set aside.

Heat a small nonstick skillet over medium heat. Add the egg, if using, in a thin layer and cook until firm. Remove. Let cool. Slice into narrow strips 1½ inches long.

To prepare the mustard dipping sauce, slowly pour the boiling water into the mustard and stir to combine. Let stand for 10 minutes. Meanwhile, crush the sesame seeds in a mortar or place in a plastic bag and crush with a rolling pin until a coarse powder forms. In a small bowl, combine the mustard, crushed sesame seeds, vinegar, sugar, soy sauce, and sesame oil. Mix well.

Place the water chestnut slices in the center of a serving platter. Arrange lettuce leaves around the water chestnuts. Place chicken, cucumber, and carrot in a spoke-like pattern on the lettuce leaves. To eat, pick up a lettuce leaf and fill with salad. Dip the lettuce packet into the mustard sauce.

*Yield: 6 rolls*

| Calories | 126 | Cholesterol | 21 mg |
|---|---|---|---|
| Fat | 4 g | Sodium | 200 mg |
| Saturated Fat | 1 g | Carbohydrate | 13 g |
| Mono | 1 g | Protein | 10 g |
| Poly | 1 g | | |

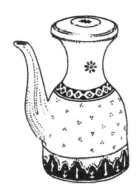

# SPICY THAI CHICKEN SALAD

## L A R B

FROM NORTHEASTERN Thailand comes this hot-and-sour chicken salad characterized by an exotic blend of flavors. Ground toasted rice provides added texture. Serve the salad on a bed of lettuce, wrap the filling in lettuce to form packages, and serve them with raw vegetables of your choice. *Larb* is wonderful as an appetizer, light lunch, or picnic food. I have substituted chicken for the ground beef usually used in Thailand. You may substitute lean ground turkey for the chicken.

The salad may be prepared one day in advance and stored, covered, in the refrigerator. Bring to room temperature before serving.

1 tablespoon long-grain rice (optional)
1 pound boneless and skinless chicken breasts and thighs, trimmed of fat,
    ground
1/3 cup fat-free low-sodium Chicken Stock (page 60)
2 tablespoons minced shallot
2 green onions, coarsely chopped
1 to 2 tablespoons fish sauce
1 stalk fresh lemon grass, bottom 6 inches only, minced
2 to 4 red chilies, seeded and minced
2 tablespoons chopped mint leaves
3 tablespoons fresh lime juice
Salt, to taste (optional)
10 romaine lettuce leaves

*Garnish*
Whole mint leaves
Lime wedges
Tomato wedges
Cucumber slices

Heat a small dry skillet over medium heat. Add the rice. Cook, stirring frequently to prevent burning, until the rice is light brown, 4 to 5 minutes. Remove from the heat. Let cool to room temperature. Grind to a fine powder in a blender or spice grinder. Set aside.

Heat a 12-inch nonstick skillet over medium heat. Add the chicken and stock and cook, stirring, until the chicken is no longer pink. Remove and set aside to cool. Add the shallot, green onions, and fish sauce to the pan. Stir for 1 minute. Remove from the heat. Combine with the chicken, lemon grass, chilies, mint, ground rice (if using), and lime juice. If desired, season with salt. Arrange in the center of a lettuce leaf. Wrap the lettuce leaf around the chicken salad and eat with your fingers. Serve with whole mint leaves, lime wedges, tomato wedges, and cucumber slices.

The salad may also be arranged on lettuce leaves on a serving platter.

*Yield: 10 rolls*

| Calories | 103 | Cholesterol | 46 mg |
|---|---|---|---|
| Fat | 2 g | Sodium | 170 mg |
| Saturated Fat | 1 g | Carbohydrate | 3 g |
| Mono | 1 g | Protein | 18 g |
| Poly | 0 g | | |

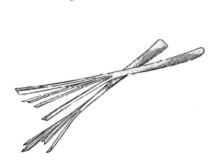

# INDIAN ROASTED EGGPLANT AND TOMATO PUREE

## BAIGAN BHARTA

YOUR TASTE buds will be awakened with this popular Indian puree. The Indian method of charring and roasting the eggplant brings out its natural flavor. I prepare the dish a day or two ahead to allow the flavors to develop in the refrigerator. Serve the puree chilled on toasted pita triangles or sesame crackers as an appetizer. In India, it is often served hot with rice.

1 to 2 Japanese eggplants (about 1½ pounds)
2 ripe medium tomatoes (about 1 pound)
2 teaspoons canola oil
1 medium onion, chopped
2 teaspoons peeled and minced fresh ginger
1 tablespoon minced garlic
1 to 2 green chilies, seeded and minced
1 teaspoon ground cumin
1 teaspoon ground coriander
½ teaspoon turmeric
¼ teaspoon red pepper powder, or to taste (optional)
Salt, to taste
2 tablespoons minced fresh coriander (cilantro)

Preheat the oven to 400 degrees. Line a baking sheet with foil.

Prick the surface of the eggplant 7 or 8 times with the tines of a fork. Over a medium gas flame, char the eggplant, turning it frequently, until all the skin has blackened and blistered. Place the eggplant on a baking sheet and bake the eggplant in the middle of the oven until very soft, 20 to 25 minutes. Cool slightly. Carefully scrape off most of the charred skin and discard. Puree the flesh to a coarse paste in a food processor or blender.

While the eggplant is cooking, peel the tomatoes. Using the tip of a knife, remove the core of each tomato. On the rounded end, cut a shallow X. Slip the tomato into boiling water for 15 to 30 seconds, or until the skin begins to pull away. Plunge the tomato into a bowl of cold water for a few seconds. Remove the tomato and pull off the skin. Cut the tomato in half crosswise. Holding cut side down over a bowl, squeeze to remove the seeds and juice. Coarsely chop the tomatoes. Set aside.

Heat the oil in a large nonstick sauté pan over medium heat. Add the onion and stir until soft. Add the ginger, garlic, chili, cumin, coriander, and turmeric. Stir for 30 seconds. Add the tomatoes and simmer for about 7 minutes, or until very soft. Add the eggplant, red pepper powder (if using), and salt. Cook, stirring often, until the mixture is a thick puree, about 5 minutes. Sprinkle with fresh coriander just before serving. Serve cold, at room temperature, or hot.

*Yield: 4 to 6 servings*

| Calories | 69 | Cholesterol | 0 mg |
| Fat | 2 g | Sodium | 9 mg |
| Saturated Fat | 0 g | Carbohydrate | 13 g |
| Mono | 1 g | Protein | 2 g |
| Poly | 1 g | | |

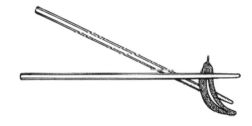

# INDIAN SPICED CHICKEN KABOBS WITH MINT-CORIANDER CHUTNEY

## MURGH TIKKA

INDIAN SPICES are combined with yogurt in a marinade for chicken kabobs. In India, the kabobs would be cooked in a clay oven called a *tandoor*. They are excellent for entertaining as they can be marinated a day ahead and put into the oven to bake just before serving. The kabobs are most attractive when served on lettuce leaves garnished with cucumber slices and lime wedges. To serve as an appetizer, place a toothpick in each morsel of meat. If serving as a main course, you may wish to leave the meat on the skewers.

If grilling, cook the chicken over medium-high heat for six to seven minutes, turning once. Immediately mist with olive oil spray. For added convenience, metal skewers can be used.

$1/2$ teaspoon salt
$1^{1}/2$ pounds boneless and skinless chicken breasts, cut into 1-inch pieces
2 tablespoons fresh lemon juice


### Yogurt Marinade
1 tablespoon peeled and chopped ginger
1 tablespoon chopped garlic
2 tablespoons plain non-fat yogurt
$1/4$ teaspoon ground cumin
$1/4$ teaspoon ground cinnamon
$1/4$ teaspoon turmeric
$1/8$ teaspoon ground cardamom
$1/8$ teaspoon ground nutmeg
$1/8$ to $1/4$ teaspoon red pepper powder
$1/2$ teaspoon paprika
2 teaspoons canola oil
Salt, to taste
Freshly ground black pepper, to taste


### Spicy Mint-Coriander Chutney
$1/4$ cup loosely packed mint leaves, coarsely chopped
$1/4$ cup loosely packed fresh coriander (cilantro) leaves, coarsely chopped

1 teaspoon peeled and chopped ginger
1/4 green chili, seeded and minced
2 teaspoons fresh lemon juice
2 tablespoons plain non-fat yogurt (optional)
Salt and freshly ground black pepper, to taste

12 bamboo skewers (6 to 8 inches), soaked in warm water for 30 minutes
Olive oil spray

### Garnish

Lettuce leaves (optional)
1 small cucumber, cut in half and thinly sliced (optional)
1 to 2 limes, cut into wedges

Sprinkle the salt over the chicken pieces. Pour the lemon juice over them. Rub the salt and lemon juice into the chicken. Set aside for 20 to 30 minutes.

In a mortar, mini processor, or blender, pound or process the ginger, garlic, and 1 tablespoon water to a paste. Combine the yogurt, cumin, cinnamon, turmeric, cardamom, nutmeg, red pepper powder, paprika, the ginger/garlic paste, and the oil in a bowl. Stir until creamy and well combined. Season with salt and pepper. Add the chicken pieces and mix thoroughly to coat. Cover and marinate in the refrigerator for 3 to 4 hours or overnight.

To prepare the Spicy Mint-Coriander Chutney, combine the mint, coriander, ginger, chili, and lemon juice in a mini food processor or blender. Process to a coarse paste. Add the yogurt, if desired, and stir until smooth. Season with salt and pepper. Place in a glass or other non-metallic container. Cover and refrigerate until ready to serve.

Preheat the oven to 350 degrees or prepare a grill to medium-high heat. Thread the chicken on the skewers, leaving about 1/2 inch between the pieces. Place the skewers on a rack over a pan and bake, turning once, for about 8 minutes, or until no longer pink in the center. Remove from the oven. Immediately mist with olive oil spray. Serve on lettuce leaves, if desired. Garnish with sliced cucumbers, if desired, and lime wedges.

*Yield: 10 to 12 appetizer or 4 dinner servings*

| | | | | |
|---|---|---|---|---|
| Calories | 57 | Cholesterol | 24 mg |
| Fat | 1 g | Sodium | 68 mg |
| Saturated Fat | 0 g | Carbohydrate | 2 g |
| Mono | 0 g | Protein | 10 g |
| Poly | 0 g | | |

# CHILLED TOFU

## HIYA-YAKKO

THE UTTER simplicity of Japanese cuisine is reflected in chilled tofu morsels garnished with green onion, shaved bonito flakes, and grated ginger. When served in individual small glass or porcelain containers, this dish is considered to be the foremost Japanese summer appetizer.

The word *yakko* is the term for food cut into squares. It is said that this shape is derived from the square of family crests on the sleeves of kimonos of the yakko, the lowest-ranking attendants in the samurai households during the Edo period.

Instant dashi powder (*dashi-no-moto*) may be used as a substitute for making your own Dashi. Dissolve a pinch of the powder in $1/4$ cup warm water.

### Sauce
$1/4$ cup low-sodium soy sauce
$1/4$ cup Dashi (page 61)
1 teaspoon mirin

1 cake (14 ounces) firm tofu, drained

### Garnishes
1 green onion, thinly sliced
2 to 3 teaspoons peeled and grated ginger, or to taste
1 tablespoon shaved bonito flakes

Combine the soy sauce, Dashi, and mirin in a small pan and cook over medium heat for 1 minute. Refrigerate for 1 hour.

Meanwhile, refrigerate the tofu for at least 1 hour. Carefully cut the tofu into 2 x 1-inch rectangles.

When ready to serve, place the tofu slices in the center of individual bowls. Garnish with green onion, ginger, and shaved bonito flakes. Pour the sauce over the tofu and serve immediately.

| Calories | 79 | Cholesterol | 1 mg |
|---|---|---|---|
| Fat | 4 g | Sodium | 273 mg |
| Saturated Fat | 1 g | Carbohydrate | 3 g |
| Mono | 1 g | Protein | 9 g |
| Poly | 2 g | | |

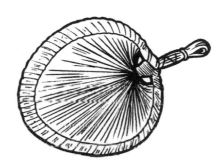

# HAND-WRAPPED SUSHI

## NIGIRI-ZUSHI

OVALS OF vinegared rice are topped with fish or shrimp in this delicacy taught to me by Kei Uchikawa, chef for the Consul General of Japan in Chicago, Tomoyuki Abe, and his wife, Motoko. Chef Uchikawa says it is of utmost importance to use impeccably fresh sushi-quality fish and seafood and to assemble the sushi just before serving. He suggests serving red pickled ginger and thinly sliced cucumbers with the sushi.

During a luncheon with Motoko Abe, Chef Uchikawa served the sushi arranged on individual lacquer trays garnished with chrysanthemum leaves. He topped the rice balls with pieces of thinly sliced raw sushi-quality tuna and red snapper, grilled eel, cooked sea scallops and shrimps, blanched cucumber, and shredded omelet. For ease in preparation, I have proposed less perishable thinly sliced smoked Nova Scotia salmon. You may use sushi-quality tuna or other seafood of your choice. Serve with pickled ginger, wasabi horseradish, and soy sauce if desired.

> 1$^1$/$_2$ tablespoons wasabi powder
> Cold water sprinkled with rice vinegar
> 2 cups freshly cooked Vinegared Rice for Sushi (recipe follows)
> $^1$/$_2$ pound thinly sliced smoked Nova Scotia salmon, sushi-quality thinly sliced
>     raw tuna, or cooked shrimp

> ***Accompaniments***
> 1 English or hothouse cucumber, cut lengthwise in half, thinly sliced
> Red pickled ginger
> Soy sauce (optional)

Mix the wasabi to a paste with 1$^1$/$_2$ tablespoons cold water. Set aside to rest for 15 minutes.

Wet your hands with the cold vinegar water to prevent the rice from sticking to your hands. Divide the rice into 30 balls, about 1 tablespoon each. Spread a small amount of the wasabi paste down the center of each piece of fish. Place a 12-inch square of heavy-duty plastic wrap in your hand. Put 1 piece of fish in the center of the plastic, then put the rice on the fish. Twist the plastic wrap to make a tight ball about the size of a large walnut. Remove from the plastic and put on a plate, pressing down slightly to flatten. Arrange sushi, cucumbers, and pickled ginger decoratively on a serving plate. Serve with an individual bowl of soy sauce, for dipping, if desired.

*Yield: 30 pieces*

| | | | |
|---|---|---|---|
| Calories | 31 | Cholesterol | 1 mg |
| Fat | 0 g | Sodium | 116 mg |
| Saturated Fat | 0 g | Carbohydrate | 5 g |
| Mono | 0 g | Protein | 2 g |
| Poly | 0 g | | |

# VINEGARED RICE FOR SUSHI

COOKED SHORT-GRAIN rice (cooked in kombu-flavored water, if desired) mixed with vinegar, sugar, and salt until it is cool is used in the preparation of sushi. To keep the rice from drying out, cover the cooled rice with a damp cloth. This rice should be used shortly after it is cooked and should not be refrigerated.

> 1 cup short-grain rice
> 1 to 1¼ cups cold water
> 1 square (2 inches) dried kelp (kombu), wiped with a damp cloth (optional)
> 2 tablespoons rice vinegar
> 2 tablespoons sugar
> 1 teaspoon sea or kosher salt, or to taste
> 2 teaspoons mirin (optional)

Put the rice in a container and add water to cover by 2 inches. Rub the grains together between the palms of your hands until the water becomes cloudy. Pour the rice in a strainer to drain. Repeat the washing procedure 3 to 5 times, or until the water is almost clear. Drain thoroughly. Place the rice, water, and kombu, if using, in a heavy 2-quart saucepan that has a tight-fitting lid. Let the rice soak for 30 minutes.

Cook the rice, covered, over medium heat until the water starts to boil. Turn the heat to high and let the water boil, as the cover bounces up and down, 4 to 5 minutes. A white, starchy liquid will bubble from under the cover. When this bubbling stops, reduce the heat to medium-low and continue to cook for 8 to 10 minutes, or until all the water has been absorbed. Do not lift the cover during cooking. Turn off the heat and let the rice steam for 15 to 20 minutes.

Combine the vinegar, sugar, salt, and mirin, if using, in a small bowl.

Transfer the cooked rice to a large shallow wooden or other non-metallic container. Using a flat wooden spoon, spread the hot rice into a thin layer. Toss the rice with the wooden paddle while fanning it with a fan or piece of cardboard. During tossing, sprinkle the dressing on the rice. Because rice varies, be careful not use so much dressing that the rice becomes mushy. The rice is ready to use when it has cooled to near room temperature.

*Yield: 2 to 2½ cups*

| Calories | 136 | Cholesterol | 0 mg |
|---|---|---|---|
| Fat | 0 g | Sodium | 355 mg |
| Saturated Fat | 0 g | Carbohydrate | 31 g |
| Mono | 0 g | Protein | 2 g |
| Poly | 0 g | | |

# EASY INDIAN SPICED CHICKEN KABOBS

FOR BUSY days, bottled *tikka* paste purchased in Indian grocery stores can be a great time-saver. Serve the kabobs with Mint-Coriander Chutney (page 237).

2 to 3 tablespoons bottled tikka paste
6 to 8 tablespoons plain non-fat yogurt
1½ teaspoons minced garlic
1½ teaspoons peeled and minced ginger
¼ to ½ teaspoon red pepper powder, or to taste
1½ pounds boneless and skinless chicken breasts, cut into 1-inch pieces
12 bamboo skewers (6 to 8 inches), soaked in warm water for 30 minutes
Olive oil spray

### Garnish
Lettuce leaves (optional)
1 small cucumber, cut in half and thinly sliced (optional)
2 to 3 limes, cut into wedges

Combine the paste, 6 tablespoons of the yogurt, garlic, ginger, and red pepper powder in a bowl. The mixture should be a thick paste. If not, add more yogurt. Mix well. Add the chicken pieces to the yogurt mixture. Mix thoroughly to coat. Cover and marinate in the refrigerator for 3 to 4 hours or overnight.

Preheat the oven to 350 degrees or prepare a grill to medium-high heat.

Thread the chicken on the skewers leaving about ½ inch between the pieces. Place the skewers on a rack over a pan and bake for about 8 minutes, or until no longer pink in the center, turning once. Remove from the oven. Immediately mist with olive oil spray. Serve on lettuce leaves, if desired. Garnish with sliced cucumbers, if desired, and lime wedges.

*Yield: 10 to 12 appetizer or 4 to 6 dinner servings*

| | | | |
|---|---|---|---|
| Calories | 50 | Cholesterol | 24 mg |
| Fat | 1 g | Sodium | 23 mg |
| Saturated Fat | 0 g | Carbohydrate | 0 g |
| Mono | 0 g | Protein | 9 g |
| Poly | 0 g | | |

# SOUPS

CHILLED ORANGE, CARROT, AND GINGER SOUP

INDONESIAN CHICKEN SOUP, JAVANESE STYLE (*Soto Ayam Jawa*)

THAI HOT AND SPICY SHRIMP SOUP

RED SNAPPER AND WATERCRESS SOUP

MISO SOUP (*Miso-Shiru*)

HEARTY MISO STEW (*Tori Miso-Shiru*)

SOBA AND CHICKEN IN BROTH (*Tori Nanban Soba*)

CHICKEN STOCK

BASIC JAPANESE SOUP STOCK (*Dashi*)

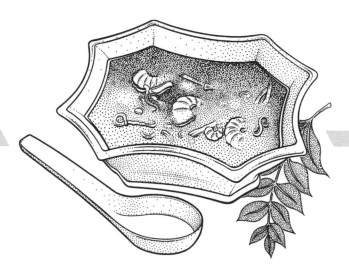

# Soups

A LIGHT piquant broth at the start of a meal lifts the winter doldrums as much as it dispels a summer swelter, all the while whetting the appetite for the next course. You'll find Japanese Dashi soup stock and Chicken Stock versatile bases for entrees and for embellishing with sliced mushrooms, a dab of miso, and/or greens such as fresh coriander. You can also have fun with these soups. For an East-West presentation, serve Chilled Orange, Carrot, and Ginger Soup or Thai Hot and Spicy Shrimp Soup in a martini glass. When serving Soba and Chicken in Broth, advise your guests to show their enjoyment by emulating the Japanese custom of slurping their noodles. If you are looking for an entree soup, look no further than Hearty Miso Stew.

# CHILLED ORANGE, CARROT, AND GINGER SOUP

THIS CONTEMPORARY combination of pureed carrots and orange juice with an accent of ginger is a cool starter for a summer luncheon or dinner. Serve the soup Hawaiian style, in a chilled martini glass, top it with a dollop of yogurt, and garnish with mint leaves.

The soup may be prepared and refrigerated one to two days ahead. Garnish when serving.

1 teaspoon olive oil
1/3 cup coarsely chopped onion
1 tablespoon peeled and coarsely chopped fresh ginger
1 pound carrots, sliced (about 4 cups)
2 teaspoons grated orange zest
3 cups fat-free low-sodium Chicken Stock (page 60)
About 1 1/2 cups fresh orange juice
3/4 teaspoon ground cinnamon
Salt and white pepper, to taste
1/3 cup plain non-fat yogurt, lightly beaten (optional)
Fresh mint leaves, for garnish

Heat the oil in a nonstick saucepan over medium heat. Add the onion, ginger, carrots, and orange zest. Sauté until the onion is translucent. Add the stock. Bring to a boil. Reduce the heat and simmer, covered, for 20 to 30 minutes, or until the carrots are tender.

Remove and puree the mixture in a blender. Return the mixture to the saucepan and add enough orange juice to produce a slightly thick consistency. Bring the soup to a simmer and cook for 2 to 3 minutes. Add the cinnamon. Season with salt and white pepper. Cover and chill thoroughly.

When serving, ladle into individual glass bowls or martini glasses. Top with a spoonful of yogurt, if desired. Garnish with fresh mint leaves.

*Yield: 4 servings*

| Calories | 125 | Cholesterol | 0 mg |
|---|---|---|---|
| Fat | 2 g | Sodium | 292 mg |
| Saturated Fat | 0 g | Carbohydrate | 24 g |
| Mono | 1 g | Protein | 6 g |
| Poly | 0 g | | |

# INDONESIAN CHICKEN SOUP, JAVANESE STYLE

## SOTO AYAM JAWA

JOELINA SOEJONO, wife of Soejono Soerjoatmodjo, Consul General of Indonesia in Chicago, showed me how she prepares this Indonesian favorite. Many versions exist throughout the country. She made it Javanese style. She serves a fiery green chili sambal as a side dish to allow each guest to spice up the soup to his or her taste.

Joelina used a whole chicken, but I have substituted skinned split chicken breasts with the bone attached and chicken thighs to lower the fat content yet have the extra flavor you get from the bones. She thinly sliced a potato and deep-fried it until golden and crisp. For ease of preparation, I have substituted baked potato chips. Candlenuts (*kemiri*), native to Indonesia, have been replaced with macadamia nuts. Daun salam, an Indonesian laurel leaf, has been replaced with a bay leaf.

2 ounces bean threads, soaked in warm water for 20 minutes and drained
3 macadamia nuts, chopped (optional)
3 cloves garlic, chopped
3 shallots, chopped
2 teaspoons turmeric
1 tablespoon canola oil
5 cups fat-free low-sodium Chicken Stock (page 60)
1½ pounds boneless and skinless chicken breasts
4 skinned chicken thighs, trimmed of fat
1 slice ginger, the size of a quarter, smashed
1 slice galangal, the size of a quarter, smashed
1 stalk lemon grass, bottom 6 inches only, smashed
1 bay leaf, crushed
Salt, to taste

### Green Chili Sambal
15 long green chilies
1 shallot, thinly sliced
1 teaspoon canola oil

### Accompaniments
1½ cups fresh bean sprouts, blanched
2 hard-boiled eggs, cut into eighths (optional)

2 green onions, green parts only, thinly sliced, or a combination of thinly sliced
   green onion and chopped celery leaves
3 tablespoons Crisp Roasted Shallots (page 275), optional
1/2 cup baked low-fat potato chips, broken into bite-size pieces

2 limes, cut into wedges

Bring 3 quarts of water to a boil. Add the drained bean threads and simmer for 1 minute, or until the noodles are just tender. Drain and set aside.

In a mortar, mini processor, or blender, pound or process the macadamia nuts to a powder. Add the garlic, shallots, and turmeric and pound or process to a paste. Heat the oil in a small nonstick skillet over medium-low heat. Add the paste mixture and cook, stirring. When the paste thickens, add 1/4 cup of the stock and continue to cook until a thick paste has formed. Set aside. (The paste mixture must cook for 2 to 3 minutes to allow the flavors to release.)

Heat the remaining stock in a large pot. Add the chicken breasts and thighs, the ginger, galangal, lemon grass, bay leaf, and the paste mixture. Bring to a boil. Reduce the heat and simmer, stirring occasionally, until the chicken is done, 20 to 25 minutes. Skim off the foam from top of stock during cooking. Remove the chicken and let cool.

Remove the meat from the bones. Shred the meat into strips about 1/8 inch wide and 1 to 1 1/2 inches long. Set aside. Season the soup with salt. If the soup has reduced, add enough water to make 5 cups. Strain. Bring to a boil.

Meanwhile, prepare the sambal. Combine the chilies, shallot, and oil in a mortar, mini processor, or blender and pound or process to a coarse paste. (If necessary, add 1 to 2 teaspoons water.)

To serve, place half of the shredded chicken, half of the bean threads, and half of the bean sprouts in a soup tureen. Ladle boiling broth over the chicken. Gently slide the hard-boiled eggs, if using, into the tureen. Scatter the green onions and the roasted shallots, if using, over the top. Serve the remaining chicken, bean sprouts, bean threads, and the potato chips in separate serving containers. Let guests add the accompaniments to their individual bowls to taste. Serve with lime wedges and a side dish of Green Chili Sambal, to be added if a spicier soup is desired.

*Yield: 4 to 6 servings*

| | | | |
|---|---|---|---|
| Calories | 321 | Cholesterol | 81 mg |
| Fat | 10 g | Sodium | 383 mg |
| Saturated Fat | 2 g | Carbohydrate | 25 g |
| Mono | 4 g | Protein | 34 g |
| Poly | 2 g | | |

# THAI HOT AND SPICY SHRIMP SOUP

THIS SOUP was inspired by Josef Budde, Executive Chef at the Grand Hyatt in Hong Kong. It is one of the most popular soups in Thailand. It is rich in contrasting tastes, and theoretically there should be an even balance between the hot and tart flavors, but you can increase or decrease the amount of chilies and lime juice to taste. If the straw mushrooms are large, cut them in half. Serve as a soup course or over rice for a complete meal.

2 stalks lemon grass
4 cups fat-free low-sodium Chicken Stock (page 60)
2 to 4 serrano or jalapeño chilies, seeds removed and cut into thin rings
3 kaffir lime leaves or $1/2$ teaspoon grated lime zest
1 can (15 ounces) straw mushrooms, drained
12 medium shrimp, shelled, deveined, and cut in half
3 tablespoons fresh lime juice
1 to 2 tablespoons fish sauce, or to taste
$1/2$ teaspoon white pepper
2 tablespoons chopped fresh coriander (cilantro) leaves

Cut the lemon grass into thirds. Bruise the bottom with the side of a knife to release the flavors.

Heat the stock in a saucepan. Add the lemon grass, chilies, and kaffir lime leaves. Simmer for about 5 minutes. Add the straw mushrooms and shrimp and cook for 2 to 3 minutes, or until the shrimp is pink and opaque. Remove and discard the lemon grass and kaffir lime leaves. Stir in the lime juice, fish sauce, and pepper. Garnish with the coriander and serve hot.

*Yield: 4 to 6 servings*

| | | | |
|---|---|---|---|
| Calories | 54 | Cholesterol | 21 mg |
| Fat | 1 g | Sodium | 696 mg |
| Saturated Fat | 0 g | Carbohydrate | 6 g |
| Mono | 0 g | Protein | 8 g |
| Poly | 0 g | | |

# RED SNAPPER AND WATERCRESS SOUP

FOR TYLUN Pang, the Executive Chef of the Westin in Maui, this soup is like "mom's chicken soup." It was made often by his Chinese grandmother, who prepared it with a local fish, menpachi, and *warabi*, fern shoots from the mountains. He says menpachi is rarely served in restaurants because it's a bony fish and very difficult to eat. When chopsticks are used and the fish is picked off the bone Chinese style, though, it is quite a delicacy. Today, Chef Pang relishes this soup as "real comfort food for my mind as well as my body." It brings back childhood memories of family trips to the mountains to pick the ferns and fishing trips for the menpachi. He suggests substituting red snapper for the menpachi and watercress for the fern shoots.

1 whole red snapper scaled and gutted with head on (about 2 pounds)
6 Chinese dried black mushrooms, soaked in hot water, about 20 minutes, stems
   removed
1/2 small red onion, cut into 1/4-inch slices
3 medium ripe tomatoes, cut into quarters
About 2 1/2 cups boiling water
6 medium shrimp, shells on
14 watercress sprigs, long stems removed
Sea salt, to taste
4 ounces tofu, drained and cut into 1-inch cubes

Cut the snapper in half or into pieces just to fit into a 4-quart saucepan. Do not remove the skin. Cut the mushrooms into quarters. Place the onion and tomatoes in the pan. Add the water and bring to a boil. Add the red snapper and mushrooms and simmer over low heat for 5 to 7 minutes, or until the fish is almost cooked. Add the shrimp and simmer until the shrimp is pink and the fish is white and opaque. The liquid should just cover the ingredients. Add watercress and cook until wilted, 20 to 30 seconds. Season with the salt. Remove from the heat. To serve, place 3 to 4 tofu cubes in each bowl. Spoon the hot soup over the tofu.

*Yield: 6 to 8 servings*

| | | | |
|---|---|---|---|
| Calories | 162 | Cholesterol | 52 mg |
| Fat | 3 g | Sodium | 71 mg |
| Saturated Fat | 1 g | Carbohydrate | 5 g |
| Mono | 1 g | Protein | 28 g |
| Poly | 1 g | | |

# MISO SOUP

## MISO - SHIRU

A TRADITIONAL Japanese breakfast would not be complete without Miso Soup and rice, fish, and pickles. Heartier versions of the soup are also served at lunch and dinner. One of the most common styles includes tofu, seaweed, and green onions. Other combinations are daikon, spinach, and seven-spice powder; potato, Chinese or napa cabbage, and lemon zest; and bite-size pieces of chicken, mushrooms, and green onions. There are no set rules regarding ingredients, except to avoid overpowering the soup by adding too many of them. No matter what ingredients you use, the method of preparation is always the same. The vegetables are first cooked in the dashi, then dissolved miso is added. Do not let the miso boil or it will lose its flavor.

Two common types of miso are *shiro-miso*, sweet and white, and *inaka-miso*, red and salty. Use about one tablespoon of miso per cup of dashi, adjusting the amount according to the saltiness of the miso. Try blending red and white miso for new flavors.

For best results, purchase good quality miso produced by a Japanese maker. The amount of salt in different kinds of miso varies widely. It is possible to purchase reduced-salt versions.

3¹/₂ cups Dashi (page 61)
3¹/₂ tablespoons Japanese white *miso*, or to taste
4 to 6 shiitake mushrooms, caps thinly sliced
¹/₂ cake (about 6 ounces) tofu, drained and cut into ¹/₂-inch cubes
3 green onions, thinly sliced
Dash of Japanese pepper powder (optional)

Heat the Dashi in a medium saucepan over medium heat. Place the miso in a small bowl, add a little Dashi, and stir to dissolve the miso. Set aside. Add the shiitakes to the saucepan and simmer until cooked, about 3 minutes. Gently add the tofu. When the tofu is hot, add the dissolved miso to the stock. Stir to dissolve. Bring to a simmer and cook for 30 seconds. Do not boil. Remove from the heat. Garnish with green onions and Japanese pepper powder, if desired. Serve immediately.

*Yield: 4 servings*

| | | | |
|---|---|---|---|
| Calories | 116 | Cholesterol | 1 mg |
| Fat | 5 g | Sodium | 564 mg |
| Saturated Fat | 1 g | Carbohydrate | 9 g |
| Mono | 1 g | Protein | 10 g |
| Poly | 3 g | | |

# HEARTY MISO STEW

## TORI MISO-SHIRU

MY FRIEND Akemi Ueki, who is from Yokohama, makes this robust winter soup with vegetables, tofu, and chicken united by miso. She says it is difficult to give an exact amount of miso because the saltiness of the miso varies with the maker. Do not boil after adding the miso because the taste will deteriorate. If Japanese taro is unavailable, substitute two small potatoes.

2 teaspoons canola oil
$1/2$ pound boneless and skinless chicken breasts, cut into bite-size pieces
5 small Japanese taros, peeled and cut into $1/2$-inch slices
2 small carrots, peeled, cut on the diagonal into $1/2$-inch slices
1 piece (2 inches) daikon, peeled, quartered, and cut into $1/2$-inch slices
4 cups Dashi (page 61)
3 to 4 tablespoons white miso, or to taste
3 to 4 shiitake mushrooms, stemmed and quartered
3 green onions, cut on the diagonal into 1-inch slices
1 cake (14 ounces) tofu, drained and cut into $1/2$-inch cubes
Japanese seven-spice powder (optional)

Heat a heavy nonstick saucepan over medium heat. Add the oil and heat it. Add the chicken and cook just until the meat begins to change color. Add the taros, carrots, and daikon. Stir for 2 minutes. Add Dashi to cover and bring to a boil. Reduce the heat to medium-low. Simmer for 15 to 20 minutes, or until the vegetables are tender. Skim to remove any foam from the surface. Place the miso in a small bowl. Add a little Dashi to the miso and stir to dissolve. Add the dissolved miso to the stew. Add 1 cup water, the mushrooms, green onions, and tofu. Stir to heat. Do not let the stew come to a boil. Serve. Let guests add seven-spice powder to taste.

*Yield: 4 servings*

| | | | |
|---|---|---|---|
| Calories | 363 | Cholesterol | 35 mg |
| Fat | 13 g | Sodium | 550 mg |
| Saturated Fat | 2 g | Carbohydrate | 32 g |
| Mono | 4 g | Protein | 32 g |
| Poly | 6 g | | |

# SOBA AND CHICKEN IN BROTH

## TORI NANBAN SOBA

KEI UCHIKAWA, chef for the Consul General of Japan in Chicago, Tomoyuki Abe, and his wife, Motoko Abe, prepared this simple one-pot dish for me. He simmered chicken, spinach, and green onions in Dashi. To serve, he placed cooked soba (buckwheat noodles) in the center of a deep bowl and carefully arranged the chicken and vegetables over the noodles, topping them with delicate yellow shreds of cooked egg omelet, an embellishment that I have omitted here.

In Japan, it is customary to drink the broth directly from your soup bowl. Japanese people usually make slurping sounds when eating the noodles—a sign of appreciation that also helps to cool the noodles down.

I have reduced the amount of soy sauce for American tastes, but Motoko says Japanese would use four to five tablespoons of soy sauce in this soup. She suggests that you provide extra soy sauce to allow your guests to add more if they like.

> 4 to 5 cups Dashi (page 61)
> 1 tablespoon sugar
> 1 to 2 tablespoons low-sodium soy sauce
> 1 pound boneless and skinless chicken breasts, cut into $3/4 \times 2$-inch strips
> 12 to 16 fresh spinach leaves
> 6 to 8 green onions, halved and sliced thin lengthwise into 2-inch lengths
> 1 package (13.7 ounces) dried soba (buckwheat noodles) or $1 1/4$ pounds fresh
>   soba
> Japanese pepper powder, to taste

Combine the Dashi, sugar, and soy sauce in a saucepan over medium heat. Bring to a gentle boil. Add the chicken and simmer for 2 to 3 minutes, or until done and no longer pink in the center. Skim to remove any foam from the surface. Add the spinach and green onions. Simmer for 1 minute.

Meanwhile, bring 4 quarts of water to a boil in a large pot over high heat. Separate the noodles and drop them into the boiling water, stirring once or twice. When the water begins to boil over, add 1 cup of cold water. Repeat twice. Continue to cook for 3 to 4 minutes after the second addition of water. The noodles should be cooked but still quite firm. Drain in a colander. Rinse with cold water, rubbing vigorously with your hands to remove all surface starch. If using fresh soba, blanch the noodles rapidly in boiling water for 10 to 15 seconds. Drain thoroughly.

To reheat the noodles, put them in a strainer in individual portions and reheat in boiling water. Place the noodles in the center of deep individual bowls. Ladle hot broth over the noodles. Arrange pieces of chicken and green onion over the noodles. Serve immediately. Season with Japanese pepper powder. Eat with chopsticks.

*Yield: 6 to 8 servings*

| | | | |
|---|---|---|---|
| Calories | 254 | Cholesterol | 38 mg |
| Fat | 3 g | Sodium | 143 mg |
| Saturated Fat | 0 g | Carbohydrate | 38 g |
| Mono | 1 g | Protein | 18 g |
| Poly | 0 g | | |

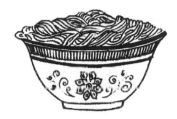

# CHICKEN STOCK

DEFATTED, LOW-SODIUM chicken stock is indispensable in light cooking. It is used for stir-fried dishes, entrees, sauces, and dressings to replace oil as well as in soups. I like to prepare a large quantity at a time. I pour it into ice cube trays. When the stock has frozen solid, I remove the cubes of stock and put them in plastic bags. Two cubes are equal to about a quarter of a cup. I then have stock immediately at hand.

When making stock, never let your pot come to a full boil.

    3 to 5 pounds chicken wings, backs, and/or necks
    2 small stalks celery with leaves
    1 large onion, quartered
    2 to 3 cloves garlic, crushed
    2 slices peeled fresh ginger, crushed
    10 black peppercorns

Rinse the chicken. Drain. Place all the ingredients in a large pan. Add water to cover by 1 inch. Heat over medium-high heat until the mixture begins to boil. Reduce the heat. Simmer the stock without boiling over low heat for 3 hours or longer, skimming the foam from surface. Remove from the heat and let the stock stand until it is cool enough to touch. Strain in a large fine-mesh strainer and cool to room temperature. Discard the solids.

Refrigerate the stock overnight, or until the fat has congealed on top. Remove the fat and discard. Ladle the stock into small freezer containers or ice cube trays. Freeze.

*Yield: About 10 cups*

Nutritional content for chicken stock is not precise enough for analysis. There are negligible calories, traces of fat, cholesterol, sodium, carbohydrates, and protein.

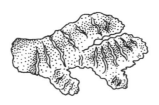

# BASIC JAPANESE SOUP STOCK

## DASHI

*DASHI*, MADE from bonito flakes and kombu (dried kelp), has a clean, refreshing taste of the sea. Used as a base for many dishes, dashi provides Japanese cooking with its unique flavor. Use good-quality kombu and bonito flakes (*katsuo-bushi*) because the quality of your soup or entree depends on the quality of the kombu and bonito flakes used in the dashi.

Instead of making it from scratch, you may choose to use instant dashi, called dashi-no-moto, as many Japanese housewives do today. However, nothing compares to the elegant subtlety of freshly made dashi. Because instant preparations vary, follow package directions when using instant dashi.

1 piece (5 × 3 inches) kombu
4 cups cold water
1/2 ounce (15 grams) dried bonito flakes

Lightly wipe the kombu clean with a lightly dampened towel. Do not wash or rinse it as its speckled surface holds the flavor. Combine the cold water and kombu in a medium sauce-pan over medium heat. Bring just to a boil. When bubbles start to rise from the bottom, remove the kelp and discard. Remove the pan from the heat. Add the bonito flakes and let sit for 1 minute. The flakes will begin to settle on the bottom of the pan. Strain the broth in a fine-meshed sieve or a sieve lined with cheesecloth. Discard the bonito.

*Yield: About 4 cups*

| | | | |
|---|---|---|---|
| Calories | 1 | Cholesterol | 1 mg |
| Fat | 0 g | Sodium | 10 mg |
| Saturated Fat | 0 g | Carbohydrate | 0 g |
| Mono | 0 g | Protein | 0 g |
| Poly | 0 g | | |

# FISH AND SEAFOOD

Grilled Mahimahi with Papaya and Maui Onion Relish

Sake-glazed Red Snapper

Japanese Glazed Salmon Steaks (*Sake no Teriyaki*)

Balinese Grilled Sea Bass in Banana Leaves

Chinese Braised Red Snapper Fillets

Steamed Red Snapper with Thai Salsa

Broiled Tuna with Mango Relish

Japanese Parchment-baked Red Snapper

Seared Ahi Tuna with Spicy Miso Vinaigrette

Indonesian Spicy Shrimp (*Belado Udang*)

Shrimp Piquant

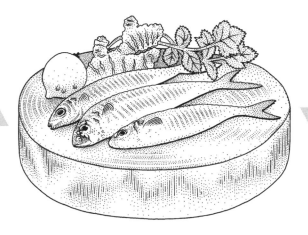

# FISH AND SEAFOOD

COOKS AROUND the Pacific Rim are dedicated to the freshness and quality of fish. To them, a fish that is still in the market at the end of the day is an old fish and is not fit for consumption. This dedication is what brought fish tanks to restaurants, where each fish is chosen straight from the tank and then prepared for cooking.

With such fine seafood, it's no wonder simple preparations abound. Here is a selection of dishes I have had the pleasure of eating, including Broiled Tuna with Mango Relish from Hawaii, Balinese Grilled Sea Bass in Banana Leaves, and Japanese Parchment-baked Red Snapper.

Besides good flavor, vibrant colors are found in such dishes as Indonesian Spicy Shrimp and the Thai-inspired Shrimp Piquant.

# GRILLED MAHIMAHI WITH PAPAYA AND MAUI ONION RELISH

HERE IS a winning combination of taste, texture, and color! This adaptation of the Hawaiian opakapaka grilled and served with a papaya and onion relish was created by George Mavrothalassitis, Executive Chef at La Mer Restaurant in the Halekulani Hotel in Honolulu. He suggested substituting mahimahi for the opakapaka. Tuna may also be substituted.

### *Papaya and Onion Relish*
1 firm ripe papaya
1/2 cup chopped Maui, Vidalia, or other sweet onion
1 tablespoon peeled and minced ginger
2 tablespoons chopped fresh coriander (cilantro) leaves
4 tablespoons fresh lime juice
1 tablespoon red wine vinegar

2 teaspoons olive oil
1 tablespoon chopped fresh coriander (cilantro) leaves
2 teaspoons minced garlic
Pinch of salt and freshly ground black pepper
4 skinless mahimahi steaks (about 6 ounces each)
4 radicchio leaves
1 medium red bell pepper, seeded and julienned

To prepare the relish, peel the papaya and cut in half. Remove the seeds and dice into 1/4-inch cubes. Combine the papaya, onion, ginger, fresh coriander, lime juice, and vinegar in a bowl. Let stand at room temperature for 30 minutes.

Combine the olive oil, coriander, garlic, salt, and pepper in a large flat glass container. Wash the fish and pat dry. Place the steaks in the marinade and let them marinate for 10 minutes.

Meanwhile, preheat a charcoal or gas grill until the fire is medium-hot.

Grill the fish about 4 minutes on each side, or until nicely browned. When done, the fish should be opaque inside.

Serve the relish on a radicchio leaf. Place the fish on top of the relish. Garnish with red bell pepper.

| Calories | 295 | Cholesterol | 149 mg |
|---|---|---|---|
| Fat | 4 g | Sodium | 190 mg |
| Saturated Fat | 1 g | Carbohydrate | 25 g |
| Mono | 2 g | Protein | 40 g |
| Poly | 1 g | | |

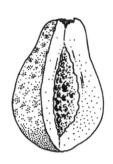

# SAKE-GLAZED RED SNAPPER

TRADITIONAL JAPANESE flavors and extremely fresh, simple ingredients are the key to the success of this fish dish, which won first place in the Hawaiian Seafood Contest for Tylun Pang, Executive Chef of the Westin, on Maui. According to him, the more attention you give the dish when basting, the better it tastes. To give the fish a final glaze, Chef Tylun put it under the broiler for about thirty to forty seconds. If you wish, you may put it in a pre-heated 400 degree oven for the final glaze.

### Sake Glaze
3 tablespoons low-sodium soy sauce
1 tablespoon plus 1 teaspoon sake
3 tablespoons mirin
2 tablespoons sugar

1 whole red snapper, scaled and gutted with head on (1¹/₂ to 2 pounds)
Salt (optional)
1 tablespoon peanut oil

### Garnish (optional)
Red pepper flakes
Julienned daikon
Julienned carrot

Combine the soy sauce, sake, mirin, and sugar in a bowl. Set aside.

Sprinkle the fish with salt on both sides, if desired. Heat a 12-inch skillet over medium heat. Add the oil. Add the fish and sauté until lightly browned on both sides. Add the glaze to the pan and heat until it begins to bubble. Baste the fish frequently until it has a thick syrupy glaze, turning the fish once. The glaze will thicken as it reduces and will coat the fish. The fish is done when the center looks opaque when tested with the tip of a knife. Sprinkle the fish with red pepper flakes and serve with a garnish of daikon and carrots, if desired.

*Yield: 3 to 4 servings*

| | | | |
|---|---|---|---|
| Calories | 241 | Cholesterol | 63 mg |
| Fat | 6 g | Sodium | 472 mg |
| Saturated Fat | 1 g | Carbohydrate | 7 g |
| Mono | 2 g | Protein | 36 g |
| Poly | 2 g | | |

# JAPANESE GLAZED SALMON STEAKS

## SAKE NO TERIYAKI

IN JAPANESE cooking, the word *"teri"* means "to shine" and *"yaki"* means to sear or broil food. Teriyaki is the sweet soy-based glaze that is applied during the last stages of grilling, broiling, or panfrying. Teriyaki sauce can be made and used immediately or refrigerated in a covered glass jar. Since it will keep in the refrigerator for six months, you may wish to prepare a larger quantity.

When Chef Kei Uchikawa prepares salmon teriyaki, he pansears it. If you wish, you may grill or broil the salmon. Salmon steaks take eight minutes per inch of thickness, so time the cooking of the fish accordingly.

*Teriyaki Sauce*
6 tablespoons low-sodium soy sauce
6 tablespoons mirin
2 teaspoons sugar

1/4 teaspoon salt
4 small salmon steaks or fillets (about 6 ounces each)
Canola oil
Japanese pickled ginger for garnish

Combine the soy sauce, mirin, and sugar in a small saucepan. Bring to a boil over medium heat, stirring until the sugar dissolves. Remove from the heat. Set aside.

Salt the fish lightly on all surfaces. Set aside for 30 minutes.

Pat the fish dry with paper towels. Heat a large nonstick skillet over medium-high heat. Brush with the oil. Add the salmon and cook on each side for 3 minutes, tilting the pan constantly to move the fish around to keep from sticking. Remove the fish from the pan. Add the teriyaki sauce. Heat until the sauce begins to bubble. Return the salmon to the pan and tilt the pan to coat the fish evenly with the sauce. Cook for about 1 minute, turning the fish once. The fish is done when the center looks opaque when tested with the tip of a knife. Remove the fish to a plate.

Continue to heat the remaining sauce, stirring constantly, until the sauce takes on a shine, about 30 seconds. Drizzle a few drops of the sauce over each steak. Serve immediately garnished with a piece of pickled ginger.

*Yield: 4 servings*

| | | | |
|---|---|---|---|
| Calories | 230 | Cholesterol | 86 mg |
| Fat | 6 g | Sodium | 1037 mg |
| Saturated Fat | 1 g | Carbohydrate | 4 g |
| Mono | 0 g | Protein | 35 g |
| Poly | 2 g | | |

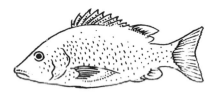

# BALINESE GRILLED SEA BASS IN BANANA LEAVES

SEA BASS fillets take on a new dimension when topped with a vividly spiced paste mixture, then wrapped in a fragrant banana leaf. Although sea bass is not traditional in Bali, where fish from the local waters would be used, I have chosen to use it because its rich, full flavor blends well with exotic flavors. Red snapper or any other firm-fleshed white fish fillets may also be used.

Fish wrapped in a banana leaf with a savory topping and baked over hot coals is among the most traditional methods of preparation in Southeast Asia. Aluminum foil can be substituted, but it provides a less dramatic presentation. Let your guests open their own packages at the table so they will be intoxicated by the perfume of the seasonings and fish.

The fillets can be wrapped several hours in advance, refrigerated, and cooked when ready to serve. You may also bake the fish in a preheated 425 degree oven.

4 thick sea bass fillets, 1 to 1½ inches, with skin (about 6 ounces each)
2 to 3 red chilies, thinly sliced
1 tablespoon peeled and minced fresh ginger
3 cloves garlic, minced
3 shallots, minced
2 tablespoons ketchup
½ teaspoon kosher salt
Freshly ground black pepper, to taste
4 squares (12 inches each) banana leaves

### Garnish
1 lime, thinly sliced
Sprigs of fresh coriander (cilantro)
1 to 2 red chilies, seeded and thinly shredded

Rinse the fillets well and pat dry. In a mortar, mini processor, or blender, pound or process the chilies, ginger, garlic, shallots, ketchup, salt, and pepper to a coarse paste, adding a little water if necessary to process. Rub the paste onto the fish.

Pour boiling water over the banana leaves to soften and prevent splitting. Place 1 fillet on each banana leaf. Garnish each fillet with the lime slices, coriander sprigs, and shredded chilies. Fold up the banana leaf, envelope style, into a neat packet. Secure the ends with metal skewers or toothpicks. Let stand for 30 minutes.

Preheat the grill until the coals are coated with a fine layer of ash.

Set the packets, seam side down, on the grill. Cover the grill and cook for about 8 minutes per inch of thickness of the fillets. Serve the fish in the banana leaf allowing each guest to unwrap his or her own package.

*Yield: 4 servings*

| | | | |
|---|---|---|---|
| Calories | 176 | Cholesterol | 70 mg |
| Fat | 3 g | Sodium | 384 mg |
| Saturated Fat | 1 g | Carbohydrate | 3 g |
| Mono | 1 g | Protein | 32 g |
| Poly | 1 g | | |

# CHINESE BRAISED RED SNAPPER FILLETS

IN THIS dish, red snapper is seared, braised in a hot-and-sour sauce with ginger, mushrooms, and onion, then attractively garnished with fresh coriander (cilantro) and red chilies. If red snapper is unavailable, substitute sea bass.

4 red snapper fillets, with skin (6 to 7 ounces each)
1/3 cup cornstarch
1 tablespoon paprika
1/2 teaspoon salt
1/4 teaspoon freshly ground black pepper
2 tablespoons canola oil
1 medium onion, cut in half and thinly sliced
2 tablespoons peeled and minced fresh ginger
1 tablespoon minced garlic
1/2 to 3/4 teaspoon red pepper powder, or to taste
6 Chinese dried black mushrooms, soaked in warm water for 20 minutes, stems
    removed, caps shredded
3 tablespoons vodka
3 tablespoons rice vinegar
1 to 2 teaspoons sugar
2 tablespoons reduced-sodium soy sauce
1 cup fat-free low-sodium fish stock or Chicken Stock (page 60)
Salt, to taste
2 tablespoons fresh coriander (cilantro) leaves
1 to 2 red chilies, seeded and julienned

Wash the fish and pat dry with paper towels. Combine the cornstarch, paprika, salt, and pepper on a dish or piece of wax paper. Dredge the fillets on the skin side in the cornstarch mixture to coat completely. Dust off the excess cornstarch. Heat the oil in a 12-inch non-stick skillet over medium-high heat until it is very hot. Gently place the fillets in the skillet, skin side down. Cook until golden brown, 2 to 3 minutes. Gently remove the fish to a platter.

Return the pan to the heat. Add the onion, ginger, garlic, and red pepper powder and cook, stirring, until the onion is translucent, about 2 to 3 minutes more. Stir in the mushrooms, vodka, vinegar, sugar, and soy sauce. Add the fish to the pan uncooked side down. Cook for about 2 minutes. Add the stock, cover, and cook until the fish is white and opaque, about 2 to 3 minutes, spooning some of the sauce over the fish occasionally. Season with salt if desired.

Place the fish on a serving platter. Pour the sauce over and around the fish. Garnish with fresh coriander and red chilies. Serve immediately.

*Yield: 4 servings*

| | | | |
|---|---|---|---|
| Calories | 368 | Cholesterol | 64 mg |
| Fat | 10 g | Sodium | 619 mg |
| Saturated Fat | 1 g | Carbohydrate | 23 g |
| Mono | 5 g | Protein | 38 g |
| Poly | 3 g | | |

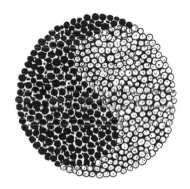

# STEAMED RED SNAPPER
# WITH THAI SALSA

A PERFECTLY steamed fresh fish is always superb. When steamed red snapper is swimming in this sauce of ripe tomatoes, avocado, tangy lime, ginger, garlic, and hot chili, the overall flavors and textures are captivating.

Azmin Ghahreman, Executive Chef of the Four Seasons Resort on Maui, adds fresh chilies during the beginning of the preparation of his salsa and completes the dish with dried red pepper flakes to round out the chili flavors.

He uses opakapaka, commonly known as crimson snapper or Hawaiian pink snapper. This fish is caught in the Hawaiian islands and is often flown to markets in the United States. Chef Azmin says red snapper can be substituted. If you prepare the salsa ahead, add the avocados just before serving and heat gently in the salsa.

### *Salsa*
1/2 teaspoon Asian sesame oil
3/4 teaspoon peanut oil
1/2 cup diced onion
1 tablespoon peeled and chopped fresh ginger
1 tablespoon chopped garlic
1/4 to 1/2 teaspoon seeded and minced red serrano chili
1 1/2 cups peeled, seeded, and diced (1/4 inch) ripe tomatoes
10 Chinese dried black mushrooms, soaked in warm water for about 20 minutes,
    stems removed, caps diced (1/4 inch)
1/4 to 1/2 cup tomato juice (optional)
1 teaspoon fish sauce
1 tablespoon fresh lime juice
2 tablespoons chopped fresh coriander (cilantro)
1 to 2 teaspoons red pepper flakes, or to taste
1 avocado, seeded, cut into 1/4-inch dice, and sprinkled with lemon juice
Salt and freshly ground black pepper, to taste

4 red snapper fillets, skin removed (4 to 6 ounces each)
Salt and freshly ground black pepper, to taste

Heat a nonstick skillet over medium heat. Add the sesame oil and peanut oil. Add the onion and sauté until translucent. Add the ginger, garlic, and chili. Stir. Cook for 30 seconds. Add the tomatoes and mushrooms and cook gently for 3 minutes, or until the tomatoes are just tender. If the salsa is too thick, add tomato juice to get the desired consistency. The mixture should be slightly thick. Stir in the fish sauce, lime juice, chopped fresh coriander, and red pepper flakes. Season with salt and pepper. Add the avocado. Stir carefully until blended and heated throughout.

Meanwhile, season the fish with salt and pepper. Steam the fish fillets over hot water until done, about 4 to 5 minutes. The fillets should be white, opaque, and tender. Place the fish in the center of a serving plate. Surround with salsa. Serve immediately.

*Yield: 4 servings*

| | | | |
|---|---|---|---|
| Calories | 264 | Cholesterol | 41 mg |
| Fat | 12 g | Sodium | 122 mg |
| Saturated Fat | 1 g | Carbohydrate | 14 g |
| Mono | 1 g | Protein | 27 g |
| Poly | 1 g | | |

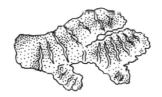

# BROILED TUNA
# WITH MANGO RELISH

IN THE elegant La Mer Restaurant in the Halekulani Hotel in Honolulu, Executive Chef George Mavrothalassitis broils opakapaka, a fish from the local waters. He suggests tuna as a substitute. When served on a bed of fresh spinach and accompanied by Mango Relish, the dish is colorful and tasty. You may grill the tuna over very hot coals if desired.

### Mango Relish
1/2 ripe mango, peeled, seeded, and diced (1/4 inch)
1/2 small red bell pepper, seeded and diced (1/4 inch)
1 1/2 teaspoons peeled and minced fresh ginger
1/2 to 1 red chili, seeded and finely chopped (optional)
1/4 cup thinly sliced red onion
1 tablespoon chopped fresh coriander (cilantro) leaves
2 tablespoons fresh lime juice
2 tablespoons fresh orange or pineapple juice
Salt and white pepper, to taste

1/4 teaspoon salt
Pinch of freshly ground black pepper
4 center-cut tuna steaks, about 3/4 inch thick (5 to 6 ounces each)
2 teaspoons minced garlic
1 tablespoon chopped fresh coriander (cilantro) leaves
2 teaspoons olive oil
12 ounces fresh spinach, washed, trimmed, and dried, for garnish

To prepare the relish, combine all of the relish ingredients in a bowl. Let stand at room temperature for 30 minutes.

Rub the salt and pepper into both sides of the fish. Prepare a marinade by mixing together the garlic, fresh coriander, and olive oil. Rub the marinade into the tuna. Allow the tuna to marinate, covered, in the refrigerator for about 30 minutes.

Preheat the broiler.

Broil the tuna 2 inches from the heat. Cook on each side for 1 1/2 minutes for rare or 2 minutes for medium. The tuna should be still rare on the inside. To test for doneness, press the tuna steaks with your finger. At medium-rare, they will yield gently. Serve on a bed of fresh spinach with the relish on the side.

| Calories | 210 | Cholesterol | 61 mg |
|---|---|---|---|
| Fat | 4 g | Sodium | 185 mg |
| Saturated Fat | 1 g | Carbohydrate | 10 g |
| Mono | 2 g | Protein | 33 g |
| Poly | 1 g | | |

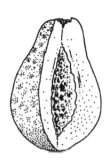

# JAPANESE PARCHMENT-BAKED
# RED SNAPPER

THIS DISH is a descendant of foods wrapped either in bamboo leaves or softened kelp, each offering its own fragrant nuance to the fish. Akemi Ueki, formerly of Yokohama but now living in Schaumburg, Illinois, uses either parchment paper or aluminum foil for her fish. She says sea bass, yellowtail, and trout are all good cooked in this manner. She tops the fish with a combination of shiitake, oyster, and cremini mushrooms, a subtle and attractive blend of mushrooms. Serve with rice, and Spinach with Toasted Sesame Seed Dressing (page 225).

Be sure to pleat the parchment sharply at each seam to make sure the packages do not open during cooking.

1/4 teaspoon salt
4 red snapper fillets (about 4 ounces each)
4 squares (12 to 14 inches) of parchment paper or heavy-duty aluminum foil
Asian sesame oil
4 tablespoons sake
4 ounces fresh shiitake, oyster mushrooms, and cremini mushrooms, cleaned,
    stems removed

### Japanese Ponzu Sauce
3 tablespoons fresh lemon juice
1 tablespoon fresh orange juice
1/4 cup low-sodium soy sauce
2 tablespoons mirin

Preheat the oven to 425 degrees.

Salt both sides of the fillet pieces and set aside for 30 minutes.

Fold each piece of parchment paper into a triangle. Open the paper and lightly brush half with the sesame oil. Arrange 1 fillet, skin side down, on the oiled portion of each of the 4 papers. Distribute one quarter of the mushrooms over each fillet. Drizzle the sake over the fish. Bring the edges of the paper together and seal the packages by crimping the parchment in a series of small, uniform folds. Place the packages on a baking sheet. Bake until the packages puff up, about 10 minutes per inch of thickness.

Meanwhile, combine the ponzu sauce ingredients. Set aside in a small serving bowl.

To serve, transfer the packets to individual serving plates. Let your guests open their own packages and top the fish with the ponzu sauce.

*Yield: 4 servings*

| | | | |
|---|---|---|---|
| Calories | 158 | Cholesterol | 42 mg |
| Fat | 2 g | Sodium | 713 mg |
| Saturated Fat | 0 g | Carbohydrate | 7 g |
| Mono | 0 g | Protein | 25 g |
| Poly | 1 g | | |

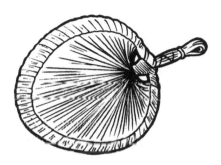

# SEARED AHI TUNA WITH
# SPICY MISO VINAIGRETTE

SUSHI-QUALITY AHI tuna is a must for this quickly seared tuna from Executive Chef Tylun Pang. He says immersing the fish in water lightens the texture and flavor, and the Spicy Miso Vinaigrette adds depth. Sushi-quality salmon may also be used.

### Spicy Miso Vinaigrette
3 tablespoons Japanese white miso
1/2 cup cider vinegar
2 tablespoons thinly sliced green onions
2 tablespoons honey
2 teaspoons peeled and finely minced ginger
2 teaspoons Asian sesame oil
2 tablespoons Chinese hot bean paste

4 center-cut blocks sushi-quality ahi tuna (3 ounces each)
Pinch salt

### Garnishes
1/4 cup julienned daikon
1/4 cup julienned carrot

In a small bowl, whisk the white miso with the vinegar until smooth. Add the remaining vinaigrette ingredients and whisk together. Set aside.

Trim and cut each piece of tuna into a block, about 2 inches across (depending on the size of the original piece). Rub salt all over the fish. Heat a pan over high flame. When it begins to smoke, quickly sear the tuna on all sides. Don't overcook. The center should remain rare. Immediately dip the tuna into iced water and pat dry.

Spoon the vinaigrette onto a serving platter. Thinly slice the ahi and arrange in the center of the vinaigrette. Garnish with daikon and carrot.

*Yield: 4 servings*

| Calories | 187 | Cholesterol | 37 mg |
|---|---|---|---|
| Fat | 4 g | Sodium | 802 mg |
| Saturated Fat | 1 g | Carbohydrate | 18 g |
| Mono | 1 g | Protein | 21 g |
| Poly | 2 g | | |

# INDONESIAN SPICY SHRIMP

## BELADO UDANG

BRIGHT RED shrimp cooked in a fiery red pepper paste is sure to spice up your meal! Joelina Soejono, who inspired this dish, is from Padang, West Sumatra. There, food is served spicy hot. She often prepares the paste mixture using only red chilies, but she says that you can alter the dish to suit your taste by combining red chilies with red bell pepper in the proportion that suits your taste. For a mild dish, use only one chili and a red pepper. The total paste mixture should be one cup.

> 1 medium red bell pepper, cored, seeded, and coarsely chopped
> 6 to 12 red chilies, seeds removed and coarsely chopped
> 1 to 2 teaspoons paprika, or to taste
> 2 tablespoons canola oil
> 2 medium shallots, thinly sliced
> 2 cloves garlic, thinly sliced
> 1 pound medium shrimp, shelled and deveined
> Salt, to taste
> Lime wedges (optional)

In a mortar, mini processor, or blender, pound or process the red bell pepper, chilies, and paprika to a paste. If necessary, add about 1 tablespoon water when processing. You should have about 1 cup of paste.

Heat a 12-inch nonstick skillet over medium heat. Add the oil and heat. Add the shallots and garlic and cook until translucent. Stir in the pepper paste and sauté for 3 to 4 minutes to release the flavors. Add water 1 tablespoon at a time if necessary to prevent the paste from sticking to the pan and burning. Stir in the shrimp and cook, stirring, until pink and opaque, 3 to 4 minutes. (If the paste becomes too thick, add water 1 tablespoon at a time.) Season with salt. Serve hot or at room temperature with rice. If desired, serve with lime wedges.

*Yield: 6 servings*

| | | | |
|---|---|---|---|
| Calories | 121 | Cholesterol | 116 mg |
| Fat | 5 g | Sodium | 133 mg |
| Saturated Fat | 1 g | Carbohydrate | 5 g |
| Mono | 3 g | Protein | 13 g |
| Poly | 2 g | | |

# SHRIMP PIQUANT

PINK SHRIMP amid red peppers, red chilies, red pepper powder, and red paprika reflect the color and fire of a brilliant sunset. This dish is inspired by Indonesian-born Executive Chef Dolf Riks of the Hilton International, Bangkok, who combines the influences of his native country with those of his adopted Thailand to produce stunning results.

The dish can be prepared ahead and reheated gently. Be sure to stir a few tablespoons of the hot dish into the yogurt to warm it before adding the yogurt gradually to the hot mixture. This will prevent it from separating. This should be done at the completion of the dish. If the dish is prepared ahead, add the yogurt just before serving.

1 tablespoon olive oil
1 large onion, diced
4 cloves garlic, finely chopped
2 tablespoons paprika
1/8 to 1/4 teaspoon red pepper flakes, or to taste
2 medium ripe tomatoes, seeded and finely diced (about 1 3/4 cups)
1 to 3 red chilies, seeded and finely chopped
2 large red bell peppers, seeded and julienned
2 tablespoons dry white wine or cognac
1 pound medium shrimp, shelled and deveined
3 tablespoons oyster-flavored sauce
Salt and freshly ground black pepper, to taste
1/4 cup plain non-fat yogurt, lightly beaten
2 tablespoons chopped fresh coriander (cilantro)

Heat the oil in a 12-inch nonstick skillet over medium heat. Add the onion and garlic. Sauté until the onion is transparent. Add the paprika and red pepper flakes. Stir for 20 seconds. Add the tomatoes. Cook, stirring occasionally, for about 2 minutes. Add the chilies, red peppers, and wine. Stir for 2 minutes. Add the shrimp and continue cooking until the shrimp is opaque, 2 to 3 minutes. Stir in the oyster-flavored sauce. Stir for about 30 seconds. Season with salt and pepper. Remove from the heat. Whisk about 2 tablespoons of the finished sauce into the yogurt. Add the warmed yogurt to the pan. Serve immediately, garnished with coriander.

*Yield: 4 to 6 servings*

| | | | |
|---|---|---|---|
| Calories | 148 | Cholesterol | 119 mg |
| Fat | 4 g | Sodium | 423 mg |
| Saturated Fat | 1 g | Carbohydrate | 14 g |
| Mono | 1 g | Protein | 16 g |
| Poly | 1 g | | |

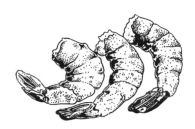

# POULTRY

Indonesian Spicy Chicken (*Ayam Bakar Kecap*)

Indonesian Chicken with Spiced Coconut Sauce (*Kalio Ayam*)

Lemon Chicken

Grilled Chicken with Balinese Barbecue Sauce

Filipino Braised Chicken (*Adobo*)

Chinese Parchment-wrapped Chicken with Gingered Vegetables

Japanese Grilled Chicken on Skewers (*Yakitori*)

Tea-smoked Turkey Breast

Chicken Satay

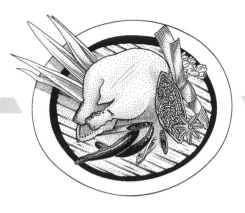

# POULTRY

THE WORLD'S universal meat is the base for an incredible variety of seasonings and marinades. Nowhere is this more true than around the Pacific, where chicken is everyday food as well as the center of celebratory feasts. Heat up your barbecue for a taste of Bali's aromatic and highly seasoned Grilled Chicken with Balinese Barbecue Sauce, Indonesia's Chicken Satay with peanut sauce, and Japan's *Yakitori*.

For elegant dining, serve aromatic Chinese Parchment-wrapped Chicken with Gingered Vegetables. Or, for a more casual approach, the Philippines' national dish, *Adobo*. Indonesian Chicken with Spiced Coconut Sauce is easy to make. Both can be prepared a day ahead. Tea-smoked Turkey Breast, served at room temperature, is perfect for a buffet.

# INDONESIAN SPICY CHICKEN

## AYAM BAKAR KECAP

THIS VIBRANTLY spiced chicken dish was inspired by Joelina Soejono, wife of Soejono Soerjoat-modjo, Consul General of Indonesia in Chicago. It is originally from Padang, West Sumatra, where the food is usually very hot and many chilies are used. She deep-fries the chicken first until it is half cooked. I sauté it until light golden brown and then proceed as she does by cooking it in the spicy paste mixture. Often she puts the chicken on a grill for a few minutes to brown it when she has finished cooking the chicken in the pan. Serve the chicken with rice.

In Indonesia, Joelina would use an aromatic (*daun salam*) leaf instead of the bay leaf. Daun salam leaves are available in some Asian grocery stores.

2 shallots, peeled and coarsely chopped

3 cloves garlic, peeled and coarsely chopped

2 red bell peppers, cored, seeded, and coarsely chopped

2 to 4 red chilies, seeded and coarsely chopped

2 tablespoons canola oil

1½ pounds boneless and skinless chicken breasts

1 bay leaf

2 to 3 slices galangal or 1 quarter-size slice ginger, smashed with the side of a knife

3 tablespoons Indonesian sweet soy sauce (*kecap manis*)

In a mini processor or blender, process the shallots, garlic, red bell peppers, and chilies to a paste. There should be about 1¾ cups. Set aside.

Heat a 12-inch nonstick skillet. Lightly spray or brush with canola oil. Add the chicken and sauté until lightly browned. (The chicken should be only half cooked.) Remove from the pan and set aside. Add the remaining oil to the pan. Add the paste mixture, bay leaf, and galangal and stir for 3 minutes to release the flavors, adding water 1 tablespoon at a time if the paste mixture is too thick and sticks to the pan. Stir in the sweet soy sauce. Return the chicken to the pan. Stir to coat the chicken on both sides with the paste mixture. Cook, turning once, until the sauce is absorbed and the chicken is fully cooked.

*Yield: 4 servings*

| | | | |
|---|---|---|---|
| Calories | 270 | Cholesterol | 73 mg |
| Fat | 10 g | Sodium | 363 mg |
| Saturated Fat | 1 g | Carbohydrate | 15 g |
| Mono | 5 g | Protein | 30 g |
| Poly | 3 g | | |

# INDONESIAN CHICKEN WITH SPICED COCONUT SAUCE

## KALIO AYAM

HERE IS another chicken dish taught to me by Joelina Soejono. This vividly spiced Padang classic is beloved among Indonesians. It is an excellent dish for entertaining as it can easily be doubled or tripled—and it tastes even better the next day when the flavors have had a chance to marry.

Joelina uses a whole chicken cut into parts because she says the bones give more flavor. I have substituted skinned chicken thighs and chicken breasts with bones to lower the fat content yet have the extra flavor the bones provide. Joelina cooks the chicken in coconut milk, which is high in cholesterol. I have substituted evaporated skim milk and unsweetened ground coconut with good results. For additional flavor, she added fresh turmeric leaves and *daun salam* leaves, both native to Indonesia. A bay leaf may be substituted for the daun salam leaf. There is no substitute for turmeric leaves. Serve this chicken with Indonesian Red Chili Sambal (page 228), Joelina's Indonesian Stir-fried Mixed Vegetables (page 180), and rice.

If you wish to use coconut milk (see page 268), cook the chicken in 3 cups thin coconut milk until tender, adding water if necessary. Add four tablespoons thick coconut milk and continue as directed.

2 teaspoons peeled and chopped fresh ginger
2 teaspoons peeled and chopped galangal
2 teaspoons chopped garlic
3 shallots, chopped
1/4 small onion, chopped
1 to 3 red chilies, seeded and chopped
2 to 3 teaspoons turmeric
2 whole split chicken breasts with bone, skinned and trimmed of fat (about 2 pounds)
4 chicken thighs, skinned and trimmed of fat (about 1 pound)
1 stalk of lemon grass, bottom 6 inches only, smashed
1 daun salam leaf or 1 bay leaf, crushed
2 cans (12 ounces each) evaporated skim milk
3 tablespoons unsweetened ground coconut, or to taste
2 kaffir lime leaves, crushed, or 1/2 teaspoon grated lemon zest
Salt, to taste

In a mortar, mini processor, or blender, pound or process the ginger, galangal, garlic, shallots, onion, chilies, and turmeric to a paste. Add 1 tablespoon water if necessary.

In a large deep saucepan, combine the chicken pieces, lemon grass, daun salam or bay leaf, the paste mixture, evaporated skim milk, and ground coconut. Add water if the chicken is not covered. Bring to a boil. Reduce the heat to a simmer and cook, stirring occasionally, until the chicken is tender, 20 to 25 minutes. If the liquid has reduced to a thick sauce, add water until it reaches the consistency of a thin cream soup. Add the kaffir lime leaves and cook for 5 minutes more. Discard the lemon grass, daun salam or bay leaf, and kaffir lime leaves. Season with salt.

*Yield: 6 servings*

| Calories | 293 | Cholesterol | 85 mg |
|---|---|---|---|
| Fat | 7 g | Sodium | 223 mg |
| Saturated Fat | 3 g | Carbohydrate | 18 g |
| Mono | 2 g | Protein | 37 g |
| Poly | 1 g | | |

# LEMON CHICKEN

TART CITRUS, a hint of chili, and sweet flavors contrast nicely with colorful red peppers and chicken served on a bed of lettuce in this Chinese dish. This is an easily prepared, do-ahead dish that can be served at room temperature or hot.

3 lemons
1½ pounds boneless and skinless chicken breasts

**Sauce Mixture**
½ cup fat-free low-sodium Chicken Stock (page 60) or water
3 tablespoons sugar
1 tablespoon cornstarch dissolved in 2 tablespoons water

3 teaspoons canola oil
1 medium red bell pepper, seeded and julienned
1 tablespoon plus 2 teaspoons peeled and julienned fresh ginger
6 Chinese dried black mushrooms, soaked in warm water for 20 minutes, stems discarded
1 to 2 red chili peppers, seeded and julienned
Salt and freshly ground black pepper, to taste
1½ cups lettuce shreds

Using a vegetable peeler, remove the zest from 1½ lemons in long strips. Cut each strip into julienne. Squeeze the 2 lemons. You should have ⅓ cup juice. Slice the remaining lemon for garnish.

Cut the chicken breasts on an angle into very thin slices, ⅛ × 1½ × 1½ inches.

To prepare the sauce, combine the stock, sugar, reserved lemon juice, and the dissolved cornstarch in a small bowl. Set aside.

Heat 1 teaspoon of the oil in a nonstick stir-fry pan or skillet over medium heat. Add the red bell pepper and stir-fry until tender to the bite, 1 to 2 minutes. Remove from the pan and set aside. Add 1 teaspoon oil to the pan. Add the ginger and stir until lightly browned, about 20 seconds. Add the chicken and stir-fry until the meat loses its pink color and is done. Remove with a slotted spoon. Set aside.

Reheat the pan and add the remaining 1 teaspoon oil. Add the mushrooms, lemon strips, and chilies. Stir until the flavors release, 20 to 30 seconds. Add the stock mixture and cook, stirring constantly, until the sugar dissolves and the sauce is shiny. Add the cooked chicken and red pepper. Toss lightly to coat and allow the flavors to mingle.

To serve, place the shredded lettuce on a platter and arrange the chicken on the lettuce. Serve hot or at room temperature.

*Yield: 4 servings*

| Calories | 275 | Cholesterol | 73 mg |
|---|---|---|---|
| Fat | 7 g | Sodium | 109 mg |
| Saturated Fat | 1 g | Carbohydrate | 25 g |
| Mono | 3 g | Protein | 30 g |
| Poly | 2 g | | |

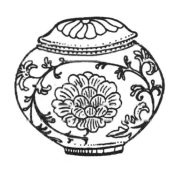

# GRILLED CHICKEN WITH BALINESE BARBECUE SAUCE

MOUTH-WATERING CHICKEN slathered with a spirited marinade brings back many fond memories of Bali, where I enjoyed it hot off the grill as well as cold while picnicking on the beach.

4 shallots, chopped
2 cloves garlic, chopped
2 to 3 red chilies, seeded and chopped
1 tablespoon peeled and chopped fresh ginger
6 macadamia nuts, chopped
3 teaspoons canola oil
3 tablespoons ketchup
1 tablespoon brown sugar
2 tablespoons low-sodium soy sauce
1½ pounds boneless and skinless chicken breasts
Lime wedges

In a mortar, blender, or mini processor, pound or process the shallots, garlic, chilies, ginger, and macadamia nuts to a coarse paste. Heat the oil in a nonstick skillet. Add the paste mixture and fry for 2 minutes, stirring. Add the ketchup, brown sugar, and soy sauce. Stir until the sugar is dissolved. Remove from the heat. Let cool.

Rub the paste mixture into the chicken and let the chicken marinate for 1 hour.

Preheat the grill.

Grill the chicken over medium coals, basting with the remaining marinade during cooking, 5 to 6 minutes on each side. The chicken is done when it is no longer pink in the center. Serve with lime wedges.

*Yield: 4 servings*

| | | | |
|---|---|---|---|
| Calories | 272 | Cholesterol | 73 mg |
| Fat | 12 g | Sodium | 482 mg |
| Saturated Fat | 2 g | Carbohydrate | 11 g |
| Mono | 8 g | Protein | 29 g |
| Poly | 2 g | | |

# FILIPINO BRAISED CHICKEN

## ADOBO

*ADOBO* IS considered the national dish of the Philippines. Its origination was dictated by the need to preserve pork during long travels. When the meat was cooked in vinegar, garlic, soy sauce, peppercorns, and other spices, it was found to keep successfully without refrigeration.

Norma Manankil, a caterer from Westmont, Illinois, who is of Filipino origin, says her adobo tastes best two days after it is cooked. Though adobo is often prepared with pork and chicken, Norma uses only chicken. She serves it with rice.

2 teaspoons canola oil
2 to 3 pounds chicken breasts and thighs, skinned
1/2 cup white vinegar
2 tablespoons low-sodium soy sauce
2 to 4 cloves garlic, minced
1/4 to 1/2 teaspoon black peppercorns
Salt and freshly ground black pepper, to taste

**Garnish (optional)**
Tomato wedges
Sprigs of parsley

Heat the oil in a nonstick saucepan over medium heat. Add the chicken and lightly brown. Add the vinegar, soy sauce, garlic, and peppercorns. Add water to just cover. Bring to a boil. Reduce the heat and simmer until the chicken is tender, 15 to 20 minutes. Remove the chicken and cook the sauce until it is reduced by half. Season with salt and pepper. Pour the sauce over the chicken. Garnish with tomato wedges and parsley sprigs, if desired, and serve.

*Yield: 6 to 8 servings*

| | | | |
|---|---|---|---|
| Calories | 112 | Cholesterol | 46 mg |
| Fat | 5 g | Sodium | 174 mg |
| Saturated Fat | 1 g | Carbohydrate | 1 g |
| Mono | 2 g | Protein | 15 g |
| Poly | 1 g | | |

# CHINESE PARCHMENT-WRAPPED CHICKEN WITH GINGERED VEGETABLES

APPETIZER-SIZE CHICKEN parcels wrapped in parchment paper and then deep-fried have been part of Chinese tradition for centuries. In my rendition, vegetable threads lend color to aromatic and delicately seasoned chicken breasts, which are wrapped in parchment and baked in the oven. They make remarkably easy, elegant fare.

Steam is trapped inside the parchment and the chicken and vegetables cook rapidly without any loss of nutrients. Be sure to pleat the parchment sharply at each seam to make sure the packages do not open during cooking.

$1^1/_2$ pounds boneless and skinless chicken breasts
2 tablespoons dry sherry or vodka
1 tablespoon low-sodium soy sauce
$^1/_4$ teaspoon sugar
4 squares (12 inches) of parchment paper or heavy-duty aluminum foil
$^3/_4$ teaspoon Asian sesame oil
1 tablespoon peeled and minced fresh ginger
2 carrots, cut into $2^1/_2$-inch-long julienne
1 medium red bell pepper, seeded and cut into thin $2^1/_2$-inch-long julienne
4 sprigs of fresh coriander (cilantro)
Salt and freshly ground black pepper, to taste

Preheat the oven to 400 degrees.

In a bowl, marinate the chicken breasts in the sherry, soy sauce, and sugar for about 30 minutes.

Fold each piece of parchment paper into a triangle. Open the triangle and lightly brush half with the sesame oil. Arrange 1 chicken breast on the oiled portion of each of the papers. Distribute one quarter of the ginger, carrots, and red pepper on top of each breast. Place a sprig of fresh coriander on top of the vegetables. Season with salt and pepper. Bring the edges of the paper together and seal the packages by crimping the parchment in a series of small, uniform folds. Place the packages on a baking sheet. Bake until the packages are puffed, about 7 to 8 minutes. To serve, transfer the packages to individual serving plates. Let your guests open their own packages.

| Calories | 199 | Cholesterol | 73 mg |
|---|---|---|---|
| Fat | 4 g | Sodium | 208 mg |
| Saturated Fat | 1 g | Carbohydrate | 9 g |
| Mono | 1 g | Protein | 28 g |
| Poly | 1 g | | |

# JAPANESE GRILLED CHICKEN ON SKEWERS

## YAKITORI

*YAKITORI* CONSIST of bite-size morsels of chicken grilled on bamboo skewers over charcoal. They are partially cooked, flavored with a sweet soy-based sauce, then put back on the grill.

Japanese chefs in the *yakitori-ya* (yakitori shops) keep their original sauce, called *"tare,"* for many years by replenishing it daily. Often it is passed down from generation to generation. Dipping the hot, cooked chicken into the pot of sauce makes it extremely flavorful.

In Tokyo, there are restaurants as well as street-side stalls that specialize in yakitori. When I am in Tokyo, I often stop in a stall to enjoy yakitori with a beer. Yakitori-ya are evening spots for businessmen who stop for a snack, a drink, and gossip on their way home from work.

You can have a yakitori party by serving the chicken kabobs with grilled skewered vegetables such as mushrooms and green peppers, a salad like Spinach with Toasted Sesame Seed Dressing (page 225), rice, and fresh fruit for dessert.

3 tablespoons sake
3 tablespoons low-sodium soy sauce
1 1/2 pounds boneless and skinless chicken breasts, cut into 1-inch pieces

**Glaze**
1/2 cup low-sodium soy sauce
1/4 cup sake
3 tablespoons mirin
1/4 cup fat-free low-sodium Chicken Stock (page 60)
2 tablespoons sugar

4 green onions, including 3 inches of the green parts, cut into 1- to 1 1/2-inch
   lengths
8 bamboo skewers, soaked in warm water for 30 minutes
Japanese pepper powder
Japanese seven-spice powder

Combine the sake and soy sauce in a large bowl. Add the chicken pieces and toss to cover. Marinate the chicken for at least 2 hours.

Combine the glaze ingredients in a small saucepan. Bring to a boil. Reduce the heat and cook, stirring, until the sauce has reduced approximately 80 percent or has thickened to a thin syrupy consistency. Set aside to cool.

Prepare a grill or preheat the broiler.

Place the chicken and green onions on the skewers, alternating the ingredients. Grill or broil for 1 to 2 minutes on one side. Brush with the glaze and grill on the other side. Repeat 2 or 3 times. Serve hot. Let your guests sprinkle the yakitori with Japanese pepper powder or seven-spice powder.

*Yield: 4 to 6 servings*

| Calories | 140 | Cholesterol | 48 mg |
|----------|-----|-------------|-------|
| Fat | 2 g | Sodium | 1187 mg |
| Saturated Fat | 1 g | Carbohydrate | 7 g |
| Mono | 1 g | Protein | 20 g |
| Poly | 0 g | | |

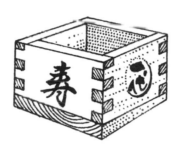

# TEA-SMOKED TURKEY BREAST

A FRAGRANT Sichuan peppercorn marinade combined with tea and sugar toasted together provides a unique and appealing flavoring for this variation of an ancient Chinese method for smoking duck. The turkey can be served warm or cold. It can be prepared up to two days ahead, and stored, well wrapped, in the refrigerator, making it ideal for entertaining. Bring to room temperature before serving. Serve it with Hawaiian Tropical Salsa (page 235).

1 tablespoon Sichuan peppercorns
4 tablespoons low-sodium soy sauce
2 tablespoons dry sherry
1 boneless and skinless turkey breast, washed and dried (about 1 1/2 pounds)

**Smoking Mixture**
3/4 cup (loosely packed) light brown sugar
3/4 cup fresh strong black tea leaves, such as Darjeeling
3/4 cup long-grain white rice

2 slices fresh ginger, smashed with the side of a knife
2 green onions, smashed with the side of a knife
1 teaspoon Asian sesame oil (optional)
1 tablespoon low-sodium soy sauce (optional)

Toast the peppercorns in an ungreased pan over medium heat until fragrant. Crush them to a coarse powder in a mortar or mini processor. Combine the crushed peppercorns, soy sauce, and sherry in a small bowl. Set aside.

Remove excess fat from the turkey. Rub the turkey on both sides with the peppercorn mixture. Let stand for 15 minutes.

Line a wok, dutch oven, or roasting pan with heavy-duty aluminum foil, allowing the foil to extend about 2 inches over the edge. Sprinkle the foil with the brown sugar, tea, and rice. Place a rack over the smoking mixture to create an air space between the tea and the pan. Line a drip pan with heavy-duty aluminum foil. Put the drip pan on the rack. Pour 1 cup water into the drip pan. Place a lightly oiled rack, such as a cake rack, over the drip pan, about 1 to 2 inches above the tea mixture. Place over medium-high heat.

Place the turkey on the rack and put the ginger and green onions on top of the turkey. Cover the wok with a foil-lined lid. The mixture will begin to smoke in about 4 minutes. Crimp the top and bottom edges of the foil together. Lower the heat to medium. Smoke the turkey until it is a rich, deep brown color, 40 to 45 minutes, or until juices run clear. The internal temperature should be 170 degrees. Turn off the heat and let the turkey stand with the cover on for 15 minutes.

Combine the sesame oil and soy sauce, if using. Remove the turkey to a serving platter. Discard the foil and tea mixture. Carve the turkey, and brush with the sesame oil–soy sauce mixture, if desired. Serve at room temperature.

*Yield: 8 to 10 appetizer servings*

| | | | |
|---|---|---|---|
| Calories | 72 | Cholesterol | 26 mg |
| Fat | 1 g | Sodium | 235 mg |
| Saturated Fat | 0 g | Carbohydrate | 2 g |
| Mono | 0 g | Protein | 12 g |
| Poly | 0 g | | |

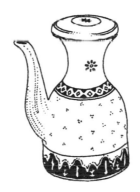

# CHICKEN SATAY

THE TANTALIZING aroma of grilled meat cooking over a charcoal fire can be sniffed through-out Southeast Asia. This all-time favorite snack sold by street vendors is served with peanut sauce. Every area of each country has its own version. Here is one of my favorites. As a variation, you may grill boneless lamb, beef, or pork.

Serve with peanut sauce and Hot-and-Sour Cucumbers (page 218) as an appetizer or as part of a meal with rice and a vegetable.

$\frac{1}{2}$ small onion, chopped
1 clove garlic, chopped
3 tablespoons low-sodium soy sauce
Juice of 1 lime
1 tablespoon brown sugar
1 teaspoon canola oil
1 pound boneless and skinless chicken breasts, cut into $2 \times \frac{1}{2}$-inch strips
Bamboo skewers, soaked in warm water for 30 minutes
Lime wedges, for garnish
Spicy Peanut Sauce (page 238)

Combine the onion, garlic, soy sauce, lime juice, brown sugar, and oil in a mini processor or blender, and process until smooth. Place the chicken in a large shallow dish and pour this marinade over the meat. Cover with plastic wrap. Marinate for 1 to 2 hours in the refrigerator, turning occasionally.

Prepare a grill or preheat the broiler.

Thread the chicken strips on skewers, two to three per skewer. Grill or broil the skewers about 4 inches from the heat until cooked through, about 3 minutes per side. Serve with lime wedges and Spicy Peanut Sauce.

*Yield: 3 to 6 servings*

| | | | |
|---|---|---|---|
| Calories | 114 | Cholesterol | 45 mg |
| Fat | 3 g | Sodium | 305 mg |
| Saturated Fat | 1 g | Carbohydrate | 4 g |
| Mono | 1 g | Protein | 18 g |
| Poly | 1 g | | |

# MEAT

Steak Kow in Oyster Sauce

Beef *Rendang*

Sichuan Stir-fried Orange Beef

Korean Marinated Grilled Beef in Lettuce Packages (*Bulgogi*)

Vietnamese Grilled Beef in Lettuce Packages with Nuoc Cham Sauce

Japanese Braised Beef, Potato, and Vegetables (*Niku Jaga*)

Mongolian Grilled Ginger Lamb Kabobs

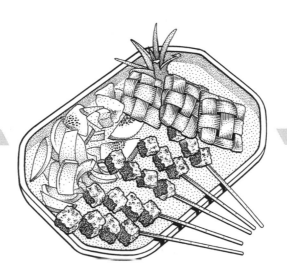

# MEAT

MEAT COOKERY in Asian cuisines sets the standard for today's recommended way of eating—small amounts of highly seasoned meat combined with sauces or vegetables and served over substantial portions of rice. Singapore's *Rendang*, a hot and spicy stew, is served with lots of rice. Japanese Braised Beef, Potato, and Vegetables is as easily prepared as it is heart-warming. And Korean *Bulgogi* is always served with rice and often accompanied by vegetables and noodle dishes. As with many of the dishes in this book, many in this chapter taste even better the next day. They are also ultimate party fare because they can be made ahead, leaving only the rice to be cooked before serving.

# STEAK KOW IN OYSTER SAUCE

MARINATED BEEF contrasts nicely with crisp snow peas in this easily prepared Chinese stir-fry. You can substitute fresh asparagus or broccoli florets for the snow peas.

1/2 pound trimmed flank steak, cut across the grain into 2 × 1 × 1/8-inch-thick
    pieces
1 tablespoon low-sodium soy sauce
1/4 teaspoon sugar
1 tablespoon cornstarch

### Oyster Sauce Mixture
4 tablespoons oyster-flavored sauce
1/2 teaspoon sugar
2 tablespoons vodka

2 teaspoons canola oil
3/4 pound snow peas, strings removed
1 teaspoon peeled and minced ginger
1 teaspoon minced garlic
5 green onions, cut into 1 1/2-inch lengths

In a bowl, combine the steak, soy sauce, sugar, and cornstarch. Let stand for 20 minutes.
Combine the oyster sauce ingredients. Set aside.
Heat a nonstick skillet or wok. Add 1 teaspoon of the oil and heat it. Add the snow peas. Stir-fry for 1 minute, or until bright green. Remove and set aside.
Add the remaining oil and heat it. Add the ginger and garlic. Cook, stirring, until fragrant, about 20 seconds. Add the steak. Stir-fry for about 3 minutes, or until the steak is done. Stir in the oyster sauce mixture. Cook and stir until it begins to bubble. Add the cooked snow peas and the green onions. Stir-fry until heated through. Serve.

*Yield: 4 servings*

| | | | |
|---|---|---|---|
| Calories | 202 | Cholesterol | 30 mg |
| Fat | 7 g | Sodium | 717 mg |
| Saturated Fat | 2 g | Carbohydrate | 13 g |
| Mono | 3 g | Protein | 19 g |
| Poly | 1 g | | |

# BEEF *RENDANG*

CHINESE TRADERS emigrated to Singapore and Malaysia about five centuries ago and married Malay wives, who were called *nonyas*. Because cooking was done by the women, the cuisine came to be called nonya. Beef *Rendang* is one of the more famous and well liked of this hot and spicy combination of Chinese and Malay cuisines. To dine in the nonya style, serve the rendang with a heaping bowl of rice, crisp cool cucumber slices, and sweet pineapple wedges.

The *rempah*, or spice paste mixture, used in this recipe is characteristic of the cuisine and imparts many interesting nuances to the dish. The spice paste mixture can be made in larger quantities and frozen for future use. I have substituted evaporated skim milk, coconut flavoring, and cornstarch for the traditional coconut milk, to produce a low-fat version without losing any of the characteristic flavor. Since coconut flavorings vary, you may have to adjust the amount used in this recipe.

The dish tastes even better the next day when the flavors have had a chance to marry. It can be easily doubled or tripled, making it an ideal dish for entertaining. It can also be frozen. Reheat on low heat being careful not to let the dish come to a boil or the sauce may curdle.

If you prefer, replace the evaporated skim milk, coconut flavoring, and cornstarch with coconut milk.

### Spice Paste Mixture
1½ tablespoons peeled and chopped ginger

3 cloves garlic, chopped

3 to 5 chilies, seeded and chopped

2 teaspoons ground coriander

1 teaspoon turmeric

2 teaspoons paprika

1 tablespoon plus 2 teaspoons cornstarch

1 can (12 ounces) evaporated skim milk

1½ teaspoons coconut flavoring

1½ tablespoons canola oil

3 cups thinly sliced onions

1 pound sirloin or top round steak, trimmed and cut into 1-inch cubes

2 stalks of lemon grass, bottom 6 inches only, smashed with the side of a knife

1 teaspoon grated lime zest

1 teaspoon sugar

Salt, to taste

In a mortar, mini processor, or blender, pound or process the ginger, garlic, and chilies and 1 to 2 tablespoons water to a coarse paste. Add the coriander, turmeric, and paprika and combine thoroughly.

Whisk the cornstarch into the evaporated skim milk in a small bowl. Stir in $^3/_4$ teaspoon of the coconut flavoring. Set aside.

Heat the oil in a large nonstick skillet over medium heat. Add the paste mixture and cook for 3 minutes, stirring. Remove 2 teaspoons of the cooked paste and whisk it into the milk mixture. Set aside.

Add the sliced onions and 2 tablespoons water to the paste in the skillet. Cook until the onions are softened, about 5 minutes. Add the meat, lemon grass, lime zest, sugar, and remaining $^3/_4$ teaspoon of the coconut flavoring. Stir until the meat is brown on all sides. Add water just to cover. Bring to a boil. Reduce the heat, cover, and simmer, stirring occasionally, until the meat is tender, 1 to 1$^1/_2$ hours. Remove the lemon grass.

When the meat is tender, make a well in the center of the pan. Recombine the milk and cornstarch mixture. Gradually whisk the milk mixture into the cooked meat. Simmer gently, whisking for about 5 minutes to allow the flavors to blend. Do not boil. Season to taste with salt. Serve.

*Yield: 6 servings*

| | | | |
|---|---|---|---|
| Calories | 233 | Cholesterol | 45 mg |
| Fat | 7 g | Sodium | 110 mg |
| Saturated Fat | 2 g | Carbohydrate | 20 g |
| Mono | 3 g | Protein | 21 g |
| Poly | 1 g | | |

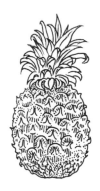

# SICHUAN STIR-FRIED ORANGE BEEF

FOUR DISTINCTIVE Sichuan ingredients—hoisin sauce, chili paste with garlic, Sichuan peppercorns, and citrus peel—make this a complex dish. In China, dried tangerine peel is used. This is often hard to find, but I like the balance of fresh orange zest with the robustness of the beef. Serve this with rice.

3/4 pound trimmed flank steak, cut across the grain into thin 1½-inch-long slices
1 tablespoon vodka
1 tablespoon low-sodium soy sauce
1 teaspoon sugar
1 teaspoon cornstarch

*Sauce Mixture*
2 tablespoons strained fresh orange juice
2 tablespoons low-sodium soy sauce
1 tablespoon hoisin sauce
½ teaspoon chili paste with garlic
3/4 teaspoon sugar

3 teaspoons canola oil
2 to 4 dried red chilies, cut in half lengthwise
1 tablespoon peeled and finely chopped fresh ginger
1 tablespoon finely chopped garlic
1 small onion, coarsely chopped
2 carrots, cut into 1½-inch-long julienne
1 large green bell pepper, cut into 1½-inch-long julienne
1 teaspoon Sichuan peppercorns toasted and finely ground
1 tablespoon finely chopped orange zest
4 green onions, cut into 1½-inch-long shreds
1 teaspoon rice vinegar
½ teaspoon Asian sesame oil
Salt, to taste

In a bowl, combine the steak, vodka, soy sauce, sugar, and cornstarch. Mix well. Let stand for 20 minutes.

Combine the sauce ingredients. Set aside.

Heat 1 teaspoon of the oil in a nonstick wok or skillet over medium heat. Add the dried chilies and stir for 10 seconds, being careful not to burn the chilies. Add the ginger, garlic, and onion and stir until the onion is translucent, about 5 minutes. Add the carrots, green pepper, and 1 tablespoon water. Stir for 2 to 3 minutes, or until crisp-tender. Remove from the pan. Heat the remaining 2 teaspoons oil. Add the beef, ground Sichuan peppercorns, and orange zest. Stir-fry until the beef is brown, about 2 minutes. Add the sauce mixture and stir-fry for 3 to 4 minutes, tossing well. Stir in the cooked carrots and green peppers and the green onions and stir until completely combined. Add the vinegar and sesame oil and salt to taste. Stir to combine. Serve right away.

*Yield: 4 to 6 servings*

| Calories | 239 | Cholesterol | 25 mg |
|---|---|---|---|
| Fat | 7 g | Sodium | 366 mg |
| Saturated Fat | 2 g | Carbohydrate | 27 g |
| Mono | 3 g | Protein | 17 g |
| Poly | 1 g | | |

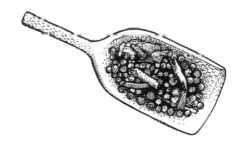

# KOREAN MARINATED GRILLED BEEF IN LETTUCE PACKAGES

## BULGOGI

*BULGOGI*, GRILLED beef cooked over an open fire, is probably one of Korea's most popular meals—and the one served at Seoul's Dae Wongak Restaurant is among the best. Its hilly parklike setting includes several thatched-roof pavilions set among ponds, stone bridges, lanterns, and large Chinese quince trees. The gazebo where I dined with friends was lit by candles and decorated with Korean antiques once used for food preparation and farming.

The small, specially designed table was close to the floor with a hole in the center housing a container of white-hot charcoal. A curved iron grill covered the charcoal. Our waitress, dressed in the traditional Korean dress, *hanbok,* grilled chopstick-size pieces of beef for us. An array of side dishes was spread on the table for us: lettuce leaves, sesame leaves, garlic, green onions, kimchi, and both raw and cooked vegetables. The waitress carefully picked up the grilled beef with chopsticks, placed it in a lettuce or sesame leaf with a sliver of raw garlic, a dab of *kochujang* (Korean chili paste), and some green onion. When bulgogi is wrapped in lettuce leaves, rice is usually served at the end, although many foreigners prefer to have it served in individual bowls during the meal. (Some Koreans enjoy their rice enclosed in the lettuce leaf.) If rice is served during the meal, you may want to place the grilled strips of meat on top of the rice and eat it with the rice. Often bulgogi is accompanied by kimchi, rice, and a salad or Korean Vermicelli, Mixed Vegetables, and Beef (page 158).

Be sure to purchase high-quality beef. For best results, have your butcher slice it into tissue-thin slices or partially freeze the beef and slice it yourself. The beef can also be sautéed in a little oil in a nonstick skillet. If desired, prepare extra marinade and dip skewered vegetables such as green peppers, white onions, carrots, and mushrooms in the marinade and then grill them.

*Marinade*
2 teaspoons sesame seeds, toasted
2 to 3 teaspoons minced garlic
3 tablespoons peeled and minced ginger
3 green onions, minced (about 1/3 cup)
3 tablespoons low-sodium soy sauce
3 tablespoons sake
1 1/2 teaspoons canola oil

1¹/₂ teaspoons sugar
Red pepper powder or freshly ground black pepper, to taste

1¹/₂ pounds lean sirloin beef, trimmed of fat, very thinly sliced, and cut into
  1-inch-long strips

### Green Onion Salad
1 teaspoon sugar
2 teaspoons sake
¹/₂ teaspoon Asian sesame oil
1 teaspoon sesame seeds, toasted (optional)
Red pepper powder, to taste
6 green onions, cut into 2-inch-long julienne

Korean chili paste or Chinese chili paste (optional)
Lettuce leaves

Combine all the marinade ingredients. Place the meat in a shallow dish. Pour the marinade over the beef and toss to coat. Cover and marinate in the refrigerator for 30 minutes to 1 hour, turning occasionally, no longer. Sirloin marinated in soy sauce for a long time tends to become tough.

Prepare a charcoal fire until the coals are white-hot.

Place the meat over the coals and grill, turning once, until it loses its pink color.

To prepare the green onion salad, combine the sugar, sake, sesame oil, sesame seeds (if using), and red pepper powder. Add the green onions and serve with the meat. (Combine the salad just before eating so that it will not become watery.)

Put a dab of chili paste on a lettuce leaf. Wrap a few pieces of beef in the lettuce. Serve with the green onion salad.

*Yield: 6 servings as a main course or 12 as an appetizer*

| Calories | 160 | Cholesterol | 65 mg |
|---|---|---|---|
| Fat | 6 g | Sodium | 137 mg |
| Saturated Fat | 2 g | Carbohydrate | 2 g |
| Mono | 3 g | Protein | 23 g |
| Poly | 1 g | | |

# VIETNAMESE GRILLED BEEF IN LETTUCE PACKAGES WITH NUOC CHAM SAUCE

YOU WILL enjoy an amazing juxtaposition of flavors and textures when you combine piquant grilled beef with cucumber, mint, fresh coriander, and slippery rice sticks. Wrap them all up in a lettuce package and dip it in a tangy and hot Vietnamese sauce for a supreme treat! Serve the lettuce packages as an appetizer, a light lunch with other dishes, or a picnic. Let your guests participate by wrapping their own packages.

1 pound lean boneless top round of beef


### Marinade
1 stalk lemon grass, bottom 6 inches only, thinly sliced
2 shallots, finely chopped
2 cloves garlic, finely chopped
1 red chili, seeded and minced
1/4 teaspoon freshly ground black pepper
1 tablespoon fish sauce
1 tablespoon fresh lime juice
1 teaspoon Asian sesame oil

Bamboo skewers, soaked in warm water for 30 minutes
1 tablespoon sesame seeds
4 ounces thin rice sticks, soaked in hot water for 20 minutes or until soft, drained
1 small cucumber, peeled, seeded, and cut into 2-inch-long julienne
12 Boston or romaine lettuce leaves
1/3 cup fresh mint leaves
Sprigs of fresh coriander
Vietnamese Nuoc Cham Sauce (page 244)

Chill the beef until just firm. Do not freeze. Slice the beef across the grain into thin 2 × 1/8-inch slices.

To prepare the marinade, in a mortar, mini processor, or blender, pound or process the lemon grass, shallots, garlic, chili, and a little water until a paste forms. Add the black pepper, fish sauce, lime juice, and sesame oil. Process until well blended. Place the beef in a shallow pan and rub the paste mixture into both sides of the beef. Let the beef marinate for at least 30 minutes or up to 8 hours in the refrigerator.

Prepare a charcoal grill or preheat the broiler.

Thread the marinated meat on the bamboo skewers and sprinkle both sides with sesame seeds. Grill or broil the beef for 1 to 2 minutes per side for rare to medium-rare. Let cool.

Meanwhile, heat 4 quarts water to a boil. Add the rice sticks and stir to separate. When the water returns to a boil, remove from the heat. Drain. Rinse with cold water. Drain again.

Place about 3 pieces of grilled beef, rice sticks, and 3 to 4 pieces of cucumber on a lettuce leaf. Put 2 or 3 mint leaves and a coriander sprig on top. Roll the lettuce leaf into a package. Repeat with the remaining leaves. Serve with the sauce.

*Yield: 12 lettuce packages*

| Calories | 122 | Cholesterol | 18 mg |
|---|---|---|---|
| Fat | 3 g | Sodium | 306 mg |
| Saturated Fat | 1 g | Carbohydrate | 14 g |
| Mono | 1 g | Protein | 11 g |
| Poly | 0 g | | |

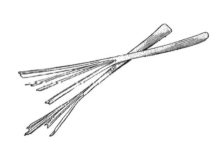

# JAPANESE BRAISED BEEF, POTATO, AND VEGETABLES

### NIKU JAGA

HERE IS a hearty family-style dish served in the home of Akemi Ueki, who is from Yokohama. A small quantity of thinly sliced beef is cooked with potatoes, carrots, and onions until almost all of the liquid has evaporated. The delicate flavor is in the vegetables seasoned with mirin, sake, and soy sauce.

Akemi says that every family has a recipe for this popular dish. She prepares it in large quantities because the flavors mellow the next day. Serve hot with rice, Japanese Smoked Salmon Salad (page 208), or Japanese pickled vegetables.

For easier slicing of the beef, partially freeze the beef before slicing or have your butcher slice it for you.

> 4 boiling potatoes (about 1½ pounds), peeled, quartered, and cut into ½-inch slices
> 2 teaspoons canola oil
> ½ pound sirloin, boneless rib or fillet, sliced paper thin
> 2 medium carrots, cut into ½-inch slices
> 2 small onions, quartered and cut into ½-inch slices
>
> *Seasonings*
> 2 to 3 tablespoons sugar
> 3 tablespoons mirin
> 1 to 2 tablespoons sake
> 3 to 4 tablespoons low-sodium soy sauce

Soak the potatoes in cold water for 15 minutes. Drain and dry with a clean dish towel.

Heat a heavy nonstick saucepan over medium heat. Add the oil and heat it. Add the meat and cook just until the meat begins to change color, then add the potatoes, carrots, and onions. Stir for 2 minutes. Add water to cover. Bring to a boil. Reduce the heat to medium-low. Skim to remove any foam. Add 1 tablespoon of the sugar, 2 tablespoons of the mirin, and 1 tablespoon of the sake. Cover and cook for 15 to 20 minutes, or until the potatoes are tender. Add 3 tablespoons of the soy sauce. Taste. Add the remaining seasonings to taste. Continue cooking until the liquid has almost evaporated, shaking the pan occasionally to prevent sticking. Serve.

| Calories | 186 | Cholesterol | 22 mg |
|---|---|---|---|
| Fat | 3 g | Sodium | 295 mg |
| Saturated Fat | 1 g | Carbohydrate | 28 g |
| Mono | 2 g | Protein | 10 g |
| Poly | 1 g | | |

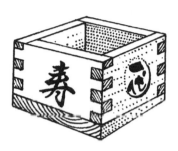

# MONGOLIAN GRILLED GINGER LAMB KABOBS

LAMB HAS played an important part in the northern Chinese cuisine since ancient times. Here, a simple mixture of ginger, soy, and honey forms a light glaze while the lamb is cooking over the hot coals.

*Marinade*
4 tablespoons low-sodium soy sauce
2 tablespoons rice wine or sake
2 tablespoons plus 1 teaspoon honey
2 teaspoons Asian sesame oil
1 clove garlic, minced
3 tablespoons peeled and minced fresh ginger
Freshly ground black pepper, to taste

1½ pounds boneless lamb, trimmed of all fat and cut into 1-inch cubes
Bamboo skewers, soaked in warm water for 30 minutes

Combine the marinade ingredients in a bowl. Add the lamb. Toss lightly to coat. Cover and let the mixture marinate overnight in the refrigerator, turning occasionally.

Prepare a charcoal grill.

Thread the lamb onto the bamboo skewers. Grill over medium-high heat for 5 to 7 minutes per side. Baste with the marinade the last few minutes of cooking. Remove from the fire. Let the lamb rest for about 5 minutes before serving.

*Yield: 6 servings*

| | | | |
|---|---|---|---|
| Calories | 155 | Cholesterol | 48 mg |
| Fat | 6 g | Sodium | 390 mg |
| Saturated Fat | 2 g | Carbohydrate | 8 g |
| Mono | 2 g | Protein | 16 g |
| Poly | 1 g | | |

# HOT POTS

JAPANESE SEAFOOD AND VEGETABLES IN BROTH (*Yosenabe*)
MONGOLIAN HOT POT
BUBBLING BEEF IN A POT (*Shabu Shabu*)
BUBBLING TOFU (*Yudofu*)

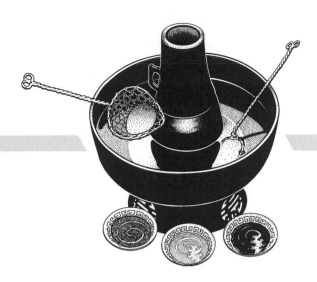

# Hot Pots

COMMUNAL tabletop cooking is one of the most social ways of entertaining. I like the way the ice is immediately broken when everyone participates in preparing dinner. Hot pot cooking in China and in Japan, where it is called *nabemono*, began because many houses did not have central heating and people could sit around the brazier to eat and to warm themselves simultaneously.

For a perfect tabletop meal, set the hot pot in the middle of the table with plates of ingredients all around. Give everyone plates and chopsticks or long-handled forks to choose the foods he or she wants to cook in the pot of hot broth. Traditionally these dishes are cooked over charcoal in an earthenware casserole or in a metal hot pot (usually of brass or copper) such as the elegant Mongolian hot pot. For authenticity the earthenware and brass pots are worth acquiring. If you choose to cook over charcoal this way, however, be sure there is plenty of ventilation in the room to dissipate the fumes and any possibility of carbon monoxide poisoning. More practical is a chafing dish or an electric skillet. Or other cookware can be set over a small portable gas burner.

All the work is done ahead of time. Ingredients are arranged on plates, and the broth and dipping sauces are prepared in advance. When your guests are seated, they dip the food into the broth to cook it, and then into the dipping sauce to season it. The broth increases in flavor as the meal progresses, and finally it, too, is consumed.

# JAPANESE SEAFOOD AND VEGETABLES IN BROTH

## YOSENABE

THIS SOUL-SATISFYING meal of exquisitely fresh fish, shellfish, and vegetables cooked in a bubbling broth is the bouillabaisse of Japan. *Yose* means to gather and *nabe* is one-pot cooking. Therefore, *yosenabe* is literally "gathering of everything." The extraordinary mélange of flavors and colors makes this dish a visual and gastronomic masterpiece.

Motoko Abe, wife of Tomoyuki Abe, Consul General of Japan, in Chicago, and author of *Quick & Easy Japanese Cooking for Everyone*, prepares the yosenabe in flameproof individual serving bowls in her kitchen. She arranges the ingredients in perfect symmetry in each bowl, then cooks them on top of the stove. She varies the dish by adding crab, clams, squid, boneless and skinless chicken breasts, and cabbage rolls.

Motoko says that in Japan yosenabe is often cooked in a *donabe*, a covered earthenware casserole that holds and conducts heat evenly and is brought to the table, and each guest helps himself. (If a donabe is not available, an attractive flameproof casserole can be used.) Sometimes guests cook their food in simmering broth at the table. Japanese specialty restaurant tables are equipped with a gas burner in the center of the table. At home, Japanese families use an alcohol or a canned-heat burner or an electric skillet.

Heat the broth in the kitchen and add the first round of ingredients in the kitchen. Bring the simmering dish to the table ready to eat. Guests can then add fish and vegetables as they like. Arrange the ingredients attractively on a platter. Let each guest choose his or her own morsels and cook them in the simmering broth. Finish the meal by adding the noodles cooked in the full-flavored broth. Serve with the dipping sauce that imparts a tangy flavor to the fresh fish and seafood.

Yosenabe is a meal in itself. Motoko also serves rice and an assortment of pickled vegetables such as Japanese Radish Salad (page 224).

*Dipping Sauce*
4 tablespoons fresh lemon juice
1 tablespoon fresh orange juice
1/4 cup low-sodium soy sauce
2 tablespoons mirin
1/8 teaspoon Japanese seven-spice powder (optional)

———

6 Chinese or napa cabbage leaves

6 ounces edible chrysanthemum leaves, watercress, or spinach, blanched

2 small carrots sliced 1/4 inch thick

**Broth**

5 cups *Dashi* (page 61)

2 tablespoons mirin

2 tablespoons low-sodium soy sauce

4 ounces shiitake or other mushrooms, cleaned and stems removed

8 green onions, cut on the diagonal into 2-inch lengths

8 ounces fillet of snapper, monkfish, or grouper, cut into bite-size pieces

12 large shrimps, shelled and deveined, with the tail on

8 ounces scallops

3 ounces bean thread (cellophane noodles), soaked in warm water for
   20 minutes and drained

To make the dipping sauce, combine the lemon juice, orange juice, soy sauce, mirin, and Japanese seven-spice powder (if using). Set aside.

Blanch the cabbage and chrysanthemum leaves separately in boiling water for 10 seconds. Remove and drain. Rinse under cold water and drain. Set aside. Blanch the carrots in boiling water for 1 to 2 minutes. Remove and drain. Rinse under cold water and drain. Set aside.

Combine the dashi, mirin, and soy sauce. Set aside.

Pour half of the broth into a flameproof casserole and bring to a boil. Reduce the heat to simmer. Add the carrots, mushrooms, and green onions and cook for 30 seconds. Add the fish pieces, one at a time. Cook for 1 minute, skimming away any foam on the surface. Add the shrimps and scallops. Cook for 30 seconds. Add the cabbage and chrysanthemum leaves. Cook for 30 seconds, adding the remaining broth or water if the broth has cooked away. Remove the casserole from the heat. Add the cellophane noodles. Cover and bring to the table piping hot. Serve in one large casserole, allowing guests to help themselves. Put the dipping sauce in small individual bowls, adding 1 tablespoon of the cooking broth to each bowl. Serve with the yosenabe.

Or arrange the remaining ingredients on a serving plate. Heat broth and cook the first round of ingredients in the kitchen. Bring the simmering casserole to the table and place on an alcohol or canned-heat burner or in an electric skillet. Invite guests to add seafood, vegetables, and noodles as they like.

| Calories | 265 | Cholesterol | 78 mg |
| Fat | 2 g | Sodium | 1006 mg |
| Saturated Fat | 0 g | Carbohydrate | 32 g |
| Mono | 0 g | Protein | 30 g |
| Poly | 0 g | | |

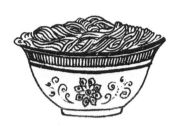

# MONGOLIAN HOT POT

THE MONGOLS used firepots as a way to cook their food during the bitterly cold winter months. The gourmets of Beijing transformed the simple firepot into the festive dish we have today. Traditionally made with lamb, it also works well with chicken or shellfish. It is an easy-to-prepare, do-ahead, elegant dinner.

There are many types of firepots or hot pots. They are made of brass, copper, or stainless steel. If you are purchasing a firepot, be sure to find one that's suitable for cooking and not merely decorative. The traditional firepot is fueled by charcoal; a chafing dish is fueled by canned heat, which is more practical, but I prefer the traditional firepot using charcoal fuel. If using charcoal, be sure you have adequate ventilation. Always fill the pot with hot broth before *adding* the charcoal. If you do not have a hot pot, use a flameproof casserole and cook over canned heat, chafing-dish style, or use an electric skillet.

Each guest gets a plate, chopsticks or a fork, a small dipper to cook ingredients in the stock, a small dish for the dipping sauce, and a soup bowl and spoon. Guests take up several pieces of meat at a time and dip them into the boiling broth. The meat cooks quickly and while it is hot, it is dipped into the dipping sauce before eating. After the meat is finished, a leafy green vegetable such as spinach or bok choy and tofu are cooked briefly in the broth, removed with chopsticks, and served to each guest. Then the bean threads are added. Finally, everyone fills his or her bowl with the tasty broth and bean threads and enjoys it as a soup.

*Dipping Sauce*
1/3 cup low-sodium soy sauce
1/3 cup fat-free low-sodium Chicken Stock (page 60)
1 tablespoon sesame seed paste or chunky peanut butter
1/4 cup dry sherry (optional)
1 tablespoon Asian sesame oil
1/4 cup chopped green onions

2 pounds tender boneless lamb; boneless and skinless chicken breasts, shredded; scallops or shrimp; or a combination
4 ounces dried bean threads (cellophane noodles), soaked in warm water for 20 minutes
2 pounds leafy green vegetables, such as spinach or bok choy, cut into bite-size pieces
1 package (14 ounces) firm tofu, drained, and cut into 1-inch squares
6 cups fat-free low-sodium Chicken Stock (page 60)

2 slices ginger, smashed with the side of a knife
2 green onions, cut in half, smashed with the side of a knife
2 green onions, finely chopped, for garnish

Combine the dipping sauce ingredients. Pour into individual dipping bowls.

For easier slicing, partially freeze the lamb until it is very firm but not solid. Slice the meat into paper-thin 3 × 1-inch strips. Drain the bean threads and cut into 4-inch lengths.

Arrange the lamb, and/or chicken and seafood on separate platters in overlapping circles. The platter should be large enough for the meat and seafood not to be overcrowded. Arrange the spinach, tofu, and bean threads on separate plates. Cover with plastic wrap and refrigerate. This may be done hours in advance.

If using charcoal, heat the charcoal outside in a charcoal grill until a white ash forms on the briquettes.

In the meantime, heat the stock, ginger, and green onions to a boil. Reduce the heat and simmer for 10 minutes. Remove the ginger and green onions and discard. Pour the boiling broth into the bowl of the firepot. With tongs, transfer the briquettes to the funnel of the firepot. Place an asbestos mat in the center of the table and set the firepot on it.

Arrange the individual platters and dipping sauce around the hot pot. Each guest cooks his or her choice of ingredients in the broth and seasons it with the dipping sauce. When the meat and vegetables are finished, ladle the broth into individual bowls. Place noodles in each bowl. Garnish each bowl with finely chopped green onion.

*Yield: 6 to 8 servings*

| | | | |
|---|---|---|---|
| Calories | 365 | Cholesterol | 77 mg |
| Fat | 15 g | Sodium | 793 mg |
| Saturated Fat | 4 g | Carbohydrate | 20 g |
| Mono | 5 g | Protein | 40 g |
| Poly | 4 g | | |

# BUBBLING BEEF IN A POT

## SHABU SHABU

*SHABU SHABU*, the name of this dish in Japanese, comes from the sound the piece of raw meat makes as you hold it in your chopsticks and swish-swish it around in a steaming broth. Paper-thin slices of beef are cooked quickly in the broth, then dipped into a lemon-based ponzu sauce. Sliced Chinese cabbage, mushrooms, and tofu are then simmered in the same liquid. Finally, bean threads (cellophane noodles) are added to the flavorful broth for a grand finale, giving you a festive one-pot meal. In Japan this is considered to be a somewhat luxurious dish served in specialty restaurants. It is also served in the home for special occasions.

Be sure to purchase high-quality beef. For best results, have your butcher slice it into tissue-thin slices across the grain.

Serve with assorted side dishes, such as Japanese Cucumber Salad (page 222), Japanese Pickled Daikon and Cucumber (page 223), and Spinach with Toasted Sesame Seed Dressing (page 225).

1½ pounds sirloin beef, very thinly sliced

¾ pound Chinese or napa cabbage, sliced into 2½-inch lengths

12 shiitake mushrooms, wiped, stems trimmed, and caps cut in half

6 ounces edible chrysanthemum leaves (see page 266) or spinach leaves, trimmed of stems

6 green onions, cut on the diagonal into 2½-inch lengths

1 cake (14 ounces) firm tofu, drained and cut into 1½-inch cubes

4 ounces bean threads (cellophane noodles), soaked in warm water for 20 minutes, drained, and cut into 6-inch lengths


### Sesame Dipping Sauce

1½ tablespoons white sesame seeds, toasted

3 tablespoons fresh lemon juice

⅓ cup low-sodium soy sauce

1 square (4 inches) piece kombu, wiped with a damp cloth and slashed in a few places to release flavors


### Japanese Ponzu Sauce

3 tablespoons fresh lemon juice

1 tablespoon fresh orange juice

¼ cup low-sodium soy sauce

2 tablespoons mirin

Finely chopped green onion, for garnish

Arrange the beef neatly on a platter in overlapping circles. The platter should be large enough so that the meat will not be overcrowded. Arrange the vegetables, tofu, and cellophane noodles on a separate platter. Cover with plastic wrap and refrigerate. This may be done hours in advance.

In a blender or mini processor, process the sesame seeds until flaky. Add the lemon juice and soy sauce. Stir to combine. Set aside. Combine the ponzu sauce ingredients. Pour into separate individual dipping bowls.

Fill a large flameproof casserole, *donabe* (see page 125), Mongolian hot pot, or electric skillet two thirds full with cold water. Add the kombu. On a stovetop burner or in the electric skillet, bring the liquid just to a boil. Remove the kombu just before the boiling point. Simmer gently for 2 to 3 minutes. Then place the casserole over an alcohol or canned-heat burner, unless you are using a Mongolian hot pot (see page 123) or an electric skillet at the table.

Arrange the platters of meat and vegetables around the hot pot. Each guest should have a plate, chopsticks or a fork, a small dish of each dipping sauce, and a soup bowl and spoon. Guests can cook their own choice of ingredients, swishing them in the simmering broth and then dipping them into dipping sauce. When the meat and vegetables are finished, add the noodles to the broth to warm them. Ladle the noodles and broth into individual bowls. Garnish each bowl with finely chopped green onion for the final course of the meal.

*Yield: 6 to 8 servings*

| Calories | 289 | Cholesterol | 49 mg |
|----------|-----|-------------|-------|
| Fat | 0 g | Sodium | 893 mg |
| Saturated Fat | 2 g | Carbohydrate | 23 g |
| Mono | 3 g | Protein | 29 g |
| Poly | 3 g | | |

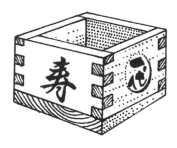

# BUBBLING TOFU

## YUDOFU

As we dined surrounded by snow-covered trees outside the Junsei Restaurant in Kyoto, *yudofu* warmed my bones. Hot tofu was simmering in a *donabe*, or earthenware pot, over charcoal, accompanied by seasoned soy sauce for dipping. This communal hot pot exemplifies the simplicity and purity of Kyoto-style cuisine. Yudofu is a dish long enjoyed by the Zen Buddhist priests and served to the general public for over three hundred years in the teahouse near the gate of the Nanzen-ji temple.

*Dipping Sauce*
$^1/_2$ cup *Dashi* (page 61)
$^1/_4$ cup low-sodium soy sauce
1 to 2 tablespoons mirin
1 tablespoon plus 1 teaspoon dried bonito flakes

1 square (4 inches) kombu, wiped with a damp cloth
2 cakes (14 ounces each) firm tofu, drained and carefully cut into 1-inch cubes

*Garnish*
3 green onions, finely sliced on the diagonal
3 teaspoons peeled and finely grated fresh ginger
1 tablespoon dried bonito flakes

To prepare the dipping sauce, combine the dashi, soy sauce, and mirin in a small saucepan over medium heat. When the mixture just reaches the boiling point, reduce the heat to a simmer. Stir in the bonito flakes. Allow to soak in the liquid for 1 to 3 seconds. Strain into another pan. Discard the bonito flakes. Set aside. Divide the dipping sauce and garnishes among small serving bowls. Set aside.

Pour 6 cups of cold water into a flameproof casserole or electric skillet. Add the kombu. Carefully slide the tofu into the cold water. Place the casserole over an alcohol or canned-heat burner at the table or place the skillet on the table. Bring the liquid just to a boil. Remove the kelp and discard. Simmer the tofu gently for 2 to 3 minutes. Do not cook too quickly or too long, or the tofu will become hard and crumble.

When the tofu is hot, gently remove it with a slotted spoon and place in individual bowls along with a little of the broth. Serve with individual bowls of hot dipping sauce. Let each guest add green onions, ginger, and bonito flakes to his bowl of dipping sauce.

*Yield: 4 to 6 servings*

| | | | |
|---|---|---|---|
| Calories | 203 | Cholesterol | 2 mg |
| Fat | 11 g | Sodium | 376 mg |
| Saturated Fat | 2 g | Carbohydrate | 7 g |
| Mono | 2 g | Protein | 22 g |
| Poly | 6 g | | |

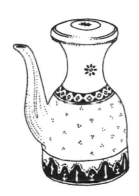

# RICE AND NOODLES

## RICE

Malaysian Rice Pilaf

Indian Spiced Rice Pilaf

Minted Saffron Rice Pilaf with Raisins and Almonds

Rice Pilaf Ring Mold Filled with Fruit and Curry Sauce

Piquant Thai Shrimp and Pineapple Fried Rice

Coconut-flavored Rice (*Nasi Lemak*)

Vegetarian Fried Rice with Macadamia Nuts

## NOODLES

Sichuan Noodles with Peanut Sauce

Spicy Rice Noodles with Vegetables, Shrimp, and Peanuts

Stir-fried Thai Noodles (*Pad Thai*)

Singapore Stir-fried Rice Noodles

Filipino Bean Threads Sautéed with Shrimp, Chicken, and Vegetables (*Pancit Guisado*)

Korean Vermicelli, Mixed Vegetables, and Beef (*Chap Chae*)

Japanese Chilled Soba Noodles in a Basket (*Zaru Soba*)

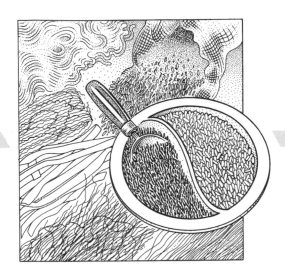

# Rice and Noodles

To Asians, food *is* rice. Perfectly steamed rice is the heart of every meal, around which all other dishes revolve. Served for breakfast, lunch, and dinner, rice is treated with great reverence. It is also important in the customs, superstitions, and religious beliefs.

Rice dishes in this chapter are enhanced by using indigenous spices and varying the preparations. (Basic rice recipes appear on pages 273–276.) You can evoke the flavors of the tropics with Rice Pilaf Ring Mold Filled with Fruit and Curry Sauce or Piquant Thai Shrimp and Pineapple Fried Rice or spice your table with the flavors of the sun with Vegetarian Fried Rice with Macadamia Nuts.

Noodles, too, are important in daily food consumption in Pacific Rim countries. They appear in many forms, from dense and pasta-like to transparent and silky. Egg noodles, wheat noodles, buckwheat noodles (soba), rice noodles, and noodles made from mung beans or potato starch provide a vast array of tastes, textures, and uses. For a perfect summer luncheon or light supper serve Japanese Chilled Soba Noodles in a Basket. If you want a little fire, try the Spicy Rice Noodles with Vegetables, Shrimp, and Peanuts, or Thailand's famed *Pad Thai*. A meal in itself is the Singapore Stir-Fried Rice Noodles, a dish that features delicately curried rice noodles with vegetables.

# RICE

# MALAYSIAN RICE PILAF

CHEF PUAN Noor Hayati Shafi of the Shangri-La Hotel in Kuala Lumpur serves this subtly flavored aromatic rice that has overtones of her north Sumatran upbringing.

1 tablespoon canola oil
1 stick (2 inches) cinnamon
1/4 teaspoon cardamom seeds
2 whole cloves
8 shallots, thinly sliced
1 tablespoon peeled and minced fresh ginger
1 clove garlic, minced
1/2 teaspoon turmeric
2 cups long-grain rice
3 3/4 cups fat-free low-sodium Chicken Stock (page 60) or water
Salt, to taste
1/4 cup golden raisins

Heat the oil in a nonstick saucepan over medium heat. Add the cinnamon, cardamom, and cloves and stir until fragrant, about 1 minute. Add the shallots, ginger, garlic, and turmeric. Stir until shallots are lightly browned, about 2 minutes.

Add the rice and stir for about 1 minute or until the grains are coated. Add the stock and salt. Bring to a boil. Reduce the heat to low. Cover the pan and cook the rice until all the liquid is absorbed, 15 to 20 minutes. Lift the lid only long enough to check that the rice has absorbed the water. Cover again. Remove from the heat. Let stand, covered, for 5 minutes. With chopsticks or a fork, fluff the rice gently. Season with salt. Sprinkle raisins over the top. Serve immediately.

*Yield: 6 to 8 servings*

| | | | |
|---|---|---|---|
| Calories | 290 | Cholesterol | 0 mg |
| Fat | 3 g | Sodium | 173 mg |
| Saturated Fat | 0 g | Carbohydrate | 58 g |
| Mono | 1 g | Protein | 7 g |
| Poly | 0 g | | |

# INDIAN SPICED RICE PILAF

IN THIS traditional Indian dish, fragrant basmati rice is combined with simple Indian spices, raisins, and toasted almonds. If using plain long-grain rice, you do not have to wash and soak the rice. I like this pilaf with grilled meat or fish.

1 cup basmati or other long-grain rice
2 teaspoons olive oil
1 medium onion, halved and thinly sliced
1 tablespoon peeled and chopped fresh ginger
$1/2$ to 1 teaspoon Madras curry powder
$3/4$ teaspoon turmeric
$1/3$ cup golden raisins
2 cups fat-free low-sodium Chicken Stock (page 60) or water
Salt, to taste
3 tablespoons slivered almonds, toasted

To wash basmati rice, place the rice in a large container. Cover with water. With your hands, swish the water around to remove the starch coating on the grains. Repeat this process until the water runs clear. Place the basmati rice in a large bowl. Add enough warm water to cover the rice by at least 1 inch. Soak the rice for at least 20 minutes to allow the grains to absorb moisture and relax before cooking. Drain the rice.

Heat the oil in a nonstick saucepan over medium heat. Add the onion and sauté, stirring, for about 2 minutes. Add the ginger, curry powder, and turmeric and stir for 20 seconds. Add the rice and raisins. Stir until the rice is almost opaque, about 3 minutes. Add the stock and salt. Bring to a boil. Lower the heat and simmer, covered, until all the water is absorbed, 15 to 20 minutes. Remove from the heat. Let stand, covered, for 5 minutes. With chopsticks or a fork, gently fluff the rice. Sprinkle almonds over the pilaf. Serve immediately.

*Yield: 4 servings*

| | | | |
|---|---|---|---|
| Calories | 273 | Cholesterol | 0 mg |
| Fat | 6 g | Sodium | 202 mg |
| Saturated Fat | 0 g | Carbohydrate | 49 g |
| Mono | 3 g | Protein | 8 g |
| Poly | 1 g | | |

# MINTED SAFFRON RICE PILAF WITH RAISINS AND ALMONDS

INDIAN SPICES and golden saffron threads join raisins, almonds, and mint in an elegant rice pilaf similar to one that I enjoyed in Madras, India. Serve this with grilled meats, poultry, seafood, or any other light dish.

1 tablespoon olive oil
1 teaspoon cardamom seeds
1 cinnamon stick, about 3 inches
2 whole cloves
1/2 cup minced onion
2 cups long-grain rice
3 1/2 cups fat-free low-sodium Chicken Stock (page 60)
1/3 cup golden raisins
1/2 to 3/4 teaspoon saffron threads, crumbled
Salt, to taste
2 tablespoons slivered almonds, toasted
1/4 cup finely chopped mint leaves

Heat the oil in a nonstick saucepan over medium heat. Add the cardamom, cinnamon, and cloves and cook, stirring, until fragrant, being careful not to burn the cardamom seeds. Add the onion and cook, stirring until translucent, 2 to 3 minutes. Add the rice and sauté for 2 to 3 minutes, making sure each grain is coated with oil.

Add the stock, raisins, saffron, and salt. Bring to a boil, stirring once. Reduce the heat to low. Cover the pan and simmer the rice until all the liquid is absorbed, 15 to 20 minutes. Lift the cover only long enough to check that the rice has absorbed the water. Cover again. Remove from the heat. Let stand, covered, for 5 minutes.

With chopsticks or a fork, gently fluff the rice. Sprinkle the almonds and mint over the rice. Serve hot.

*Yield: 6 to 8 servings*

| | | | |
|---|---|---|---|
| Calories | 231 | Cholesterol | 0 mg |
| Fat | 3 g | Sodium | 150 mg |
| Saturated Fat | 0 g | Carbohydrate | 45 g |
| Mono | 2 g | Protein | 6 g |
| Poly | 0 g | | |

# RICE PILAF RING MOLD FILLED WITH FRUIT AND CURRY SAUCE

THIS SPICED Indian rice pilaf ring filled with fresh fruits in season and topped with a delicately spiced curry sauce will be the hit of your next dinner party. Prepare the fruit ahead. Make the sauce while you cook the rice. Put it into the mold just before serving.

3/4 cup ripe pineapple chunks

1 small ripe mango, sliced

1/2 cup orange segments

1 ripe peach or pear, peeled and cut into slices

1/3 cup sweet dessert wine, such as late harvest Riesling

### Pilaf

2 teaspoons olive oil

2 medium onions, coarsely chopped

2 teaspoons minced ginger

2 cups long-grain rice

4 cups fat-free low-sodium Chicken Stock (page 60)

Salt, to taste

### Curry Sauce

1 1/2 tablespoons golden raisins

1 teaspoon cornstarch dissolved in 2 teaspoons sweet dessert wine

1/8 teaspoon Madras curry powder

2 tablespoons chopped fresh coriander (cilantro) leaves

1 tablespoon chopped unsalted dry-roasted peanuts

Combine the fruit in a bowl. Add the wine and let marinate for 1 1/2 hours. Drain, reserving the liquid. Cover and refrigerate fruit.

Heat the oil in a 4-quart nonstick saucepan. Add the onions and ginger and cook until onion is translucent, about 2 minutes. Add the rice and cook, stirring, until all the grains are coated. Add 3 1/2 cups of the stock and salt. Bring to a boil. Reduce the heat to low. Cover the pan and cook the rice until all the liquid is absorbed, 15 to 20 minutes. Rinse a ring mold in cold water. Pack the hot rice firmly into the mold. Let it rest for 5 minutes. Invert mold onto a serving platter. Unmold.

While the rice is cooking, prepare the sauce. Combine the reserved marinade, the remaining ¹/₂ cup stock and raisins in a small pan. Bring to a rolling boil over medium-high heat. Continue to cook for 2 to 3 minutes to reduce the liquid slightly. Add the curry powder. Stir. Recombine the cornstarch-wine mixture and add to the liquid in the pan. Stir until the sauce is shiny and has thickened slightly.

Arrange the fruit in the center and around the edge of the rice mold. Pour the warm sauce over the rice. Garnish with fresh coriander and peanuts. Serve immediately.

*Yield: 6 to 8 servings*

| Calories | 271 | Cholesterol | 0 mg |
|---|---|---|---|
| Fat | 2 g | Sodium | 173 mg |
| Saturated Fat | 0 g | Carbohydrate | 54 g |
| Mono | 1 g | Protein | 7 g |
| Poly | 0 g | | |

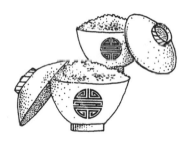

# PIQUANT THAI SHRIMP AND PINEAPPLE FRIED RICE

STIR-FRIED RICE with shrimp, refreshing pineapple, and a touch of chili is one of my family favorites. For an attractive presentation, I serve the rice in a pineapple shell. You place the cooked fried rice in a large pineapple shell and bake it in a preheated 375 degree oven until heated throughout. Garnish with red chilies and fresh coriander.

$2^1/_2$ teaspoons canola oil
3 shallots, minced
6 ounces shrimp, cooked
4 Chinese dried black mushrooms, soaked in warm water for about 20 minutes,
    stems removed, caps shredded
$^1/_2$ teaspoon grated lemon zest
2 tablespoons fish sauce
3 cups cold cooked long-grain rice
2 eggs, lightly beaten (optional)
$^3/_4$ cup bite-size pieces fresh pineapple

### Garnish
1 to 2 red chilies, seeded and finely julienned into $1^1/_2$-inch-long pieces
Fresh coriander (cilantro) leaves

Heat a large nonstick skillet or stir-fry pan. Add 1 teaspoon of the oil. Add the shallots and stir-fry for about 20 seconds. Add the shrimp, mushrooms, lemon zest, and fish sauce. Stir-fry for 30 seconds. Remove and set aside.

Add 1 teaspoon oil. Heat. Add the rice, stirring with chopsticks until thoroughly heated. Make a well in the center of the rice. Add the remaining $^1/_2$ teaspoon of oil. Add the eggs, if using, and let them set slightly. When they have a soft-scrambled consistency, start incorporating the rice in a circular fashion with chopsticks. When the rice and eggs are blended, add the shrimp mixture. Stir. Add the pineapple. Stir until thoroughly combined and heated throughout. Place on a serving platter. Garnish with red chilies and coriander leaves.

*Yield: 3 to 4 servings*

| | | | |
|---|---|---|---|
| Calories | 264 | Cholesterol | 83 mg |
| Fat | 4 g | Sodium | 443 mg |
| Saturated Fat | 1 g | Carbohydrate | 42 g |
| Mono | 2 g | Protein | 14 g |
| Poly | 1 g | | |

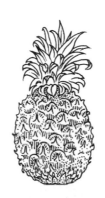

# COCONUT-FLAVORED RICE

## N A S I   L E M A K

THROUGHOUT SOUTHEAST Asia, coconut-flavored rice often accompanies sauced dishes like Beef *Rendang* (page 110) and Thai curries. It is usually prepared with coconut milk. I have used skim milk with coconut powder to give it a coconut flavor. Unsweetened coconut powder can be found in Indian grocery stores. If unavailable, grind unsweetened coconut flakes to a powder in the food processor or blender. Pandanus leaves are traditionally used in cooking the rice. I have substituted bay leaf.

2³/₄ cups skim milk
1¹/₂ cups long-grain rice
1 bay leaf
¹/₄ cup freshly grated coconut or 3 to 4 teaspoons unsweetened coconut powder
Salt, to taste

Bring the milk almost to a boil. Add the rice and bay leaf. Bring just to a boil. Reduce the heat, cover, and simmer until all the milk is absorbed, 15 to 20 minutes. Do not lift the cover during this time. At the end of this period, lift the cover long enough to check to see that all the milk has been absorbed. Cover again and remove from the heat. Let the rice rest for at least 5 minutes. With chopsticks or a fork, add the coconut and salt and fluff the rice. Serve warm.

*Yield: 4 servings*

| | | | |
|---|---|---|---|
| Calories | 330 | Cholesterol | 3 mg |
| Fat | 2 g | Sodium | 91 mg |
| Saturated Fat | 2 g | Carbohydrate | 65 g |
| Mono | 0 g | Protein | 11 g |
| Poly | 0 g | | |

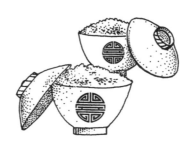

# VEGETARIAN FRIED RICE WITH MACADAMIA NUTS

A RAINBOW of colors, tastes, and textures greets you in this vegetarian fried rice inspired by Gary Strehl, Executive Chef of the Hawaii Prince Hotel in Honolulu. For a heartier dish, add cooked chicken or shrimp. The recipe makes three to four servings as a meal, more if served with other dishes.

1 teaspoon light olive oil
2 teaspoons peeled and minced fresh ginger
1 to 2 cloves garlic, minced
2 tablespoons diced onion
1 medium red bell pepper, seeded and diced
1 medium green bell pepper, seeded and diced
1/2 cup mushrooms, sliced
1 medium carrot, diced
3 cups cold cooked long-grain rice
2 to 3 tablespoons low-sodium soy sauce
1 green onion, finely sliced
2 tablespoons chopped toasted macadamia nuts

Heat the oil in a nonstick stir-fry pan over medium heat. Add the ginger and garlic. Stir-fry until fragrant, 20 to 30 seconds. Add the onion, red and green bell peppers, mushrooms, and carrot. Stir until the vegetables are crisp-tender. Remove from the pan and set aside. Add the cooked rice and stir gently in a circular motion until heated through. Add the cooked vegetables. Season to taste with the soy sauce. Stir in the green onion and macadamia nuts. Serve.

*Yield: 6 servings*

| | | | |
|---|---|---|---|
| Calories | 157 | Cholesterol | 0 mg |
| Fat | 3 g | Sodium | 182 mg |
| Saturated Fat | 0 g | Carbohydrate | 29 g |
| Mono | 2 g | Protein | 4 g |
| Poly | 0 g | | |

# SICHUAN NOODLES WITH PEANUT SAUCE

VIBRANT COLORS and vibrant flavors highlight this popular cold noodle salad, a specialty of Bruce Kraig, President of the Culinary Historians of Chicago. Crisp vegetables and chicken contrast with a spicy peanut sauce drizzled over fresh Chinese egg noodles.

This recipe can be doubled easily and prepared in advance. Arrange the noodle platter one hour before serving. Pass the peanut sauce separately or toss with the noodles when serving.

The peanut sauce tastes best if prepared at least one hour prior to serving. It will keep for one week, covered, in the refrigerator.

$^3$/$_4$ pound fresh thin Chinese egg noodles or 8 ounces dried thin noodles or
    spaghettini
1 teaspoon Asian sesame oil
1$^1$/$_2$ pounds boneless and skinless chicken breasts


***Peanut Sauce***
1 tablespoon plus 1$^1$/$_2$ teaspoons peeled and minced fresh ginger
3 teaspoons peeled and minced garlic
3 tablespoons low-sodium soy sauce
3 tablespoons rice vinegar
1$^1$/$_2$ to 2 teaspoons Chinese chili paste with garlic
$^1$/$_4$ cup reduced-fat peanut butter
1 tablespoon plus 2 teaspoons sugar
$^1$/$_4$ cup fat-free low-sodium Chicken Stock (page 60) or water

1 small cucumber, peeled, halved, seeded, and cut into thin julienne
1 red bell pepper, seeded and cut into thin julienne
2 carrots, cut into thin julienne
4 to 6 Chinese dried black mushrooms, soaked in warm water for 20 minutes,
   stems removed, caps thinly shredded (optional)
1$^1$/$_2$ cups fresh bean sprouts (optional)
2 green onions, finely sliced

Separate the fresh noodles by fluffing them with your hands. Bring 4 quarts water to a boil in a large pan. Add the noodles. When the water returns to a boil, separate the noodles with chopsticks. Test the noodles every 30 seconds until al dente. Drain immediately and refresh under cold running water. Drain again. Toss with the sesame oil. Cover and refrigerate. (If cooking dried pasta, cook according to the package directions and refresh as above.)

Heat 3 quarts of water to a boil. Add the chicken breasts and bring the water back to boiling. Reduce the heat to low and simmer for about 20 minutes, or until the meat is no longer pink in the center. Remove and let cool. Cut the chicken into 2-inch-long julienne.

To prepare the peanut sauce, in a small bowl, whisk the ginger, garlic, soy sauce, vinegar, chili paste with garlic, peanut butter, sugar, and stock until thoroughly blended. If the sauce is too thick, add more stock and blend until smooth. Transfer to a serving container. Let stand for 1 hour before serving.

Place the chilled noodles on a serving platter. Combine the cucumber, red pepper, carrots, mushrooms, and bean sprouts, if using, and half the green onions and arrange around the edge of the noodles. Place the chicken in the center. Sprinkle the remaining green onions over the chicken. Cover with plastic wrap and refrigerate until ready to serve.

Pass the peanut sauce with the salad or pour over just before serving.

*Yield: 6 to 8 servings*

| Calories | 285 | Cholesterol | 37 mg |
| Fat | 4 g | Sodium | 204 mg |
| Saturated Fat | 1 g | Carbohydrate | 43 g |
| Mono | 2 g | Protein | 20 g |
| Poly | 1 g | | |

# SPICY RICE NOODLES WITH VEGETABLES, SHRIMP, AND PEANUTS

THE LINGERING hint of lime, fish sauce, mint, and fresh coriander, along with colorful crisp fresh vegetables and shrimp pervades cold rice noodles in this Vietnamese favorite. For best flavor and texture, add the dressing just before serving.

8 ounces rice sticks (rice vermicelli), soaked in warm water for 20 minutes and
    drained
3/4 cup fresh bean sprouts
3 tablespoons rice vinegar
1/3 cup fresh lime juice
2 tablespoons plus 1 teaspoon fish sauce
1 red chili, seeded and minced (optional)
1 large clove garlic, minced
2 teaspoons sugar
Salt, to taste
1 carrot, peeled and cut into 2-inch-long julienne
1/2 cucumber, peeled, seeded, and cut into 2-inch-long julienne
8 ounces cooked medium shrimp, halved lengthwise
2 tablespoons chopped fresh mint leaves
2 tablespoons chopped fresh coriander (cilantro) leaves
2 tablespoons Crisp Roasted Shallots (page 277) (optional)
2 tablespoons coarsely chopped unsalted dry-roasted peanuts

Heat 4 quarts of water to a boil. Add the rice sticks and stir to separate. When the water returns to a boil, drain. Refresh with cold water and drain for 5 minutes, lifting occasionally to allow the noodles to dry. Blanch the bean sprouts in boiling water for 30 seconds. Drain. Refresh with cold water and drain again.

To prepare the dressing, in a small bowl, combine the rice vinegar, lime juice, fish sauce, chili, garlic, and sugar. Season with salt, if desired. Set aside.

Transfer the noodles to a large bowl. Add the rice vinegar mixture and toss well. Add the bean sprouts, carrot, cucumber, and shrimp and toss to combine. Add the mint, coriander, and shallots and toss again. Transfer to shallow bowls. Sprinkle with the peanuts. Serve at once.

| Calories | 229 | Cholesterol | 74 mg |
| Fat | 3 g | Sodium | 366 mg |
| Saturated Fat | 1 g | Carbohydrate | 39 g |
| Mono | 1 g | Protein | 13 g |
| Poly | 1 g | | |

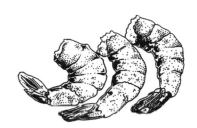

# STIR-FRIED THAI NOODLES

## PAD THAI

NOODLES PLAY an important role in Thailand, especially as a snack. Every cook in Thailand has his or her own version of this shrimp and rice noodle dish with its hot and sour garnishes.

*Pad Thai* is usually made with dried thin flat rice noodles. If unavailable, any size rice noodles may be used. Cooked chicken shreds may be used as a substitute for the shrimp.

8 ounces dried thin flat rice noodles, $1/8$ inch wide, soaked in warm water for
    20 minutes and drained
1 to 2 tablespoons light brown sugar
3 tablespoons fish sauce
2 tablespoons tomato ketchup
2 tablespoons fat-free low-sodium Chicken Stock (page 60)
1 tablespoon canola oil
1 tablespoon plus 1 teaspoon minced garlic
3 tablespoons minced shallots
12 medium shrimps, cooked
1 tablespoon red pepper powder (optional)
2 eggs, lightly beaten
$1\frac{1}{2}$ cups fresh bean sprouts
Salt, to taste

### Garnishes
$1/2$ to 1 teaspoon red pepper flakes
$1/2$ tablespoon dried shrimp, pounded or ground to a powder (optional)
1 to 2 tablespoons unsalted dry-roasted peanuts, coarsely chopped
2 green onions, finely sliced
2 tablespoons chopped fresh coriander (cilantro) leaves
2 limes, cut into wedges

Cook the rice noodles in 4 quarts of boiling water for 2 to 3 minutes, or until al dente. Drain and rinse well with cold water. Spread them on a towel to dry slightly.

Combine the brown sugar, fish sauce, ketchup, and stock in a small bowl. Set aside.

Heat the oil in a 10- to 12-inch nonstick skillet or wok. Add the garlic and shallots and fry until light brown, being careful not to burn. Add the shrimps and red pepper powder.

Stir-fry until heated through. Stir in the sauce mixture and toss to combine. Stir in the eggs and let set slightly. Stir until they reach a soft scrambled consistency. Stir in half of the noodles and toss to thoroughly incorporate them into the mixture. Add the remaining noodles and half of the bean sprouts. Season with salt. Toss until thoroughly combined and the bean sprouts are just wilted.

Place the noodle mixture on a large platter. Place the remaining bean sprouts on the side of the platter. Sprinkle the red pepper flakes, shrimp powder, peanuts, green onions, and coriander over the noodle mixture. Arrange the lime wedges around the edge of the platter and serve.

*Yield: 4 servings*

| | | | |
|---|---|---|---|
| Calories | 364 | Cholesterol | 139 mg |
| Fat | 7 g | Sodium | 697 mg |
| Saturated Fat | 2 g | Carbohydrate | 61 g |
| Mono | 3 g | Protein | 15 g |
| Poly | 2 g | | |

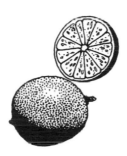

# SINGAPORE STIR-FRIED RICE NOODLES

DELICATELY CURRIED rice noodles are speckled with colorful vegetables and shrimp in a lively blend of spices and textures. Make the noodles a meal with Hot-and-Sour Cucumbers (page 220).

1 cup broccoli florets
1 tablespoon plus 1 teaspoon canola oil
1 teaspoon peeled and minced fresh ginger
1 teaspoon minced garlic
1 small carrot, cut into 1 1/2-inch-long julienne
1 small zucchini, cut into 1 1/2-inch-long julienne
1 medium red bell pepper, seeded and julienned
6 green onions, shredded into 1 1/2-inch lengths
1 to 2 red or green chilies, seeded and minced
2 teaspoons Madras curry powder, or to taste
1/2 teaspoon turmeric
1/4 teaspoon red pepper powder
1/2 pound cooked small shrimp
1 cup fresh bean sprouts
8 ounces rice sticks (rice vermicelli), soaked in warm water for 20 minutes and drained
2 tablespoons low-sodium soy sauce
1/3 cup fat-free low-sodium Chicken Stock (page 60)
Salt, to taste

### Garnish
2 tablespoons chopped dry-roasted unsalted peanuts
2 limes, cut into wedges

Blanch the broccoli in boiling water for 45 seconds, or until crisp-tender. Drain. Refresh under cold water. Drain and pat dry. Set aside.

Heat 1 teaspoon of the oil in a nonstick wok or large skillet over medium heat. Add the ginger and garlic. Stir-fry until fragrant, about 20 seconds. Add the carrot. Stir for 1 minute. Add the zucchini, broccoli, bell pepper, half of the green onions, and the chilies. Stir for 2 minutes, or until the vegetables are crisp-tender. Remove from the pan and set aside.

Add the remaining oil to the pan. Add the curry powder, turmeric, and red pepper powder. Stir for about 10 seconds, being careful not to burn. Add the remaining green onions, the shrimp, and bean sprouts and toss for about 30 seconds, or until heated. Add the rice sticks and toss to coat and heat them. When they are hot, return the vegetables to the pan. Add the soy sauce, stock, and salt. Toss gently until combined and heated. Reduce the heat to low and cook, tossing occasionally, until the liquid is absorbed, 2 to 3 minutes. Garnish with the peanuts. Serve immediately with lime wedges.

*Yield: 6 servings*

| | | | |
|---|---|---|---|
| Calories | 249 | Cholesterol | 74 mg |
| Fat | 5 g | Sodium | 315 mg |
| Saturated Fat | 1 g | Carbohydrate | 40 g |
| Mono | 2 g | Protein | 14 g |
| Poly | 1 g | | |

# FILIPINO BEAN THREADS SAUTÉED WITH SHRIMP, CHICKEN, AND VEGETABLES

### PANCIT GUISADO

NOODLES WERE introduced to the Philippines by the Chinese. Filipinos added their own flavors to make *pancit*, which is their generic term for noodle dishes. This dish, with braised bean threads tossed with chicken, shrimp, and colorful vegetables, comes from Norma Manankil, a Filipino caterer now living in Westmont, Illinois.

Twelve ounces of fresh thin Chinese egg noodles or capellini or eight ounces of thin dried egg noodles may be substituted for the bean threads. Cook according to package directions. Follow the recipe directions for bean threads when adding the cooked noodles to the dish.

8 ounces bean threads (cellophane noodles), soaked in warm water for
    20 minutes and drained
2 teaspoons canola oil
1 medium onion, quartered, thinly sliced
2 to 3 cloves garlic, minced
1/2 pound boneless and skinless chicken breasts, cut into bite-size pieces
1/2 pound small shrimp, shelled
1 1/2 cups fat-free low-sodium Chicken Stock (page 60)
1 cup thinly sliced cabbage
3 medium carrots, cut into 1 1/2-inch-long julienne (about 1 cup)
4 to 5 celery stalks, thinly cut on the diagonal (about 1 cup)
10 Chinese dried black mushrooms, soaked in warm water for 20 minutes, stems
    removed, caps julienned
10 snow peas, thinly sliced on the diagonal
2 tablespoons low-sodium soy sauce, or to taste
2 tablespoons oyster-flavored sauce, or to taste
Salt and freshly ground black pepper, to taste
2 green onions, finely sliced
Lime wedges

Cut the drained bean threads into 3-inch lengths. Set aside.

Heat 1 teaspoon of the oil in a nonstick sauté pan over medium heat. Add the onion and garlic and cook, stirring, until the onion is translucent, about 2 minutes. Add the chicken and shrimp. Stir-fry until almost done, 1 to 2 minutes. Add the stock and bring to a boil over high heat. Stir in the cabbage, carrots, celery, mushrooms, and snow peas and cook until crisp-tender, about 2 minutes. Add the bean threads. Season to taste with the soy sauce, oyster-flavored sauce, salt, and pepper. Toss the noodles to combine and simmer until heated through. Sprinkle with green onions. Serve with lime wedges.

*Yield: 6 to 8 servings*

| | | | |
|---|---|---|---|
| Calories | 225 | Cholesterol | 62 mg |
| Fat | 2 g | Sodium | 429 mg |
| Saturated Fat | 0 g | Carbohydrate | 36 g |
| Mono | 1 g | Protein | 14 g |
| Poly | 1 g | | |

# KOREAN VERMICELLI, MIXED VEGETABLES, AND BEEF

## CHAP CHAE

HERE IS a vegetable and beef stir-fry prepared with noodles made from potato and sweet potato starch. Chung Hea Han, a well-known Seoul cooking school owner and author of *Korean Cooking*, taught me this dish. She says that in Korea this is not considered a noodle dish, but a vegetable or side dish that could be served with *Bulgogi* (page 114). Korean potato starch noodles are available in Korean markets. If unavailable, use Chinese bean threads.

### Beef Marinade
1 teaspoon sesame seeds, toasted
2 tablespoons low-sodium soy sauce
1 green onion, minced
2 teaspoons minced garlic
$1/2$ teaspoon sugar
$1/2$ teaspoon Asian sesame oil (optional)

$3/4$ pound lean beef top round or sirloin, cut across the grain into 2-inch-long julienne

### Sauce Mixture
3 tablespoons low-sodium soy sauce
1 teaspoon sugar
1 teaspoon freshly ground black pepper, or to taste
1 teaspoon Asian sesame oil (optional)

8 ounces Korean potato starch noodles or bean threads

2 teaspoons canola oil
1 large carrot, cut into $1^{1}/_{2}$-inch-long julienne
1 celery stick, cut on the diagonal into thin slices
1 medium onion, quartered, thinly sliced lengthwise
1 medium zucchini, cut into $1^{1}/_{2}$-inch-long julienne
$1/2$ cup julienned bamboo shoots (about 3 ounces)

5 to 6 Chinese dried black mushrooms, soaked in warm water for about
   20 minutes, stems removed, caps julienned
Red pepper powder, to taste
3 green onions, cut into 2-inch-long julienne

Crush the sesame seeds in a mortar to a coarse powder or place in a plastic bag and crush with a rolling pin. Combine the sesame powder, soy sauce, green onion, garlic, sugar, and sesame oil, if using, in a bowl. Add the beef and marinate for 20 to 30 minutes.

To make the sauce mixture, combine the soy sauce, sugar, pepper, and sesame oil, if using, and set aside.

Bring 6 quarts of water to a boil. Add the noodles and stir until soft, barely 1 minute. Remove and immediately plunge into a colander and rinse with cold water. Drain well. Cut into 2-inch lengths with scissors. Set aside.

In a large nonstick wok or skillet, heat 1 teaspoon of the oil over medium-high heat. Add the carrot, celery, and onion. Stir-fry until almost crisp-tender, about 2 minutes. Add the zucchini and bamboo shoots and stir until the vegetables are crisp-tender. Remove and set aside on a plate.

Heat the remaining 1 teaspoon oil in the wok. Add the beef and mushrooms. Stir-fry until the meat is browned, 1 to 2 minutes. Stir in the noodles and the sauce mixture and toss for about 1 minute, or until combined. Toss in the reserved vegetables to warm. Arrange on a serving platter. Sprinkle red pepper powder over the dish. Garnish with green onion.

*Yield: 6 to 8 servings*

| | | | |
|---|---|---|---|
| Calories | 200 | Cholesterol | 24 mg |
| Fat | 3 g | Sodium | 358 mg |
| Saturated Fat | 9 g | Carbohydrate | 30 g |
| Mono | 2 g | Protein | 13 g |
| Poly | 1 g | | |

# JAPANESE CHILLED SOBA NOODLES IN A BASKET

### ZARU SOBA

DURING THE hot and humid summers, the Japanese love to eat chilled soba (buckwheat noodles), accompanied by a dipping sauce highlighted with daikon and wasabi (Japanese horseradish).

While in Tokyo, I ate in many noodle shops. One of my favorites was Kanda-Yabusoba Restaurant. To get there, you walk down a winding path through a garden to a traditional old-style Japanese house. The interior of the restaurant is understated Japanese elegance, with traditional tatami mats on the floor. Owner Yasuhiko Hotta told me that the restaurant had been in the family since the seventeenth century, and that the art of noodle making had been passed down from generation to generation. He took me into the kitchen, where I watched skilled noodle chefs hand knead the dough. Then they rolled it on ancient hand-cranked noodle-makers.

Fresh soba can be purchased in Japanese and specialty markets.

### Dipping Sauce
1½ cups *Dashi* (page 61)
¼ cup low-sodium soy sauce
1 to 2 teaspoons sugar
2 tablespoons mirin

8 ounces dried thin soba or ¾ pound fresh soba
¼ cup toasted and finely shredded nori

### Condiments
¼ cup finely chopped green onion
3 to 4 tablespoons grated daikon
1 to 2 teaspoons wasabi (Japanese horseradish) powder mixed with 1 to
    2 teaspoons cold water and set aside to rest for 15 minutes

Combine the dipping sauce ingredients in a small pan. Bring just to a boil. Remove from the heat. Set aside to cool.

Bring 2 quarts of water to a boil in a large pot over high heat. Separate the noodles and drop them into the boiling water, stirring once or twice. When the water begins to boil over, add 1 cup of cold water. Repeat twice. Lower the heat and cook until the noodles are tender, about 3 to 4 minutes. The noodles should be cooked through, but still quite firm. Drain in a colander. Rinse with cold water until completely chilled, rubbing vigorously with hands to remove all surface starch. If using fresh soba, blanch the noodles in rapidly boiling water for 10 to 15 seconds. Drain thoroughly. Rinse as above.

Place the noodles in a bamboo basket lined with a bamboo mat or on a glass plate. Sprinkle the nori over the soba. Put the dipping sauce in small individual containers. Let each guest add green onion, daikon, and a dash of wasabi to his container of dipping sauce. To eat, dip the noodles into the sauce, a few at a time. With noodles, chopsticks work far better than a fork.

*Yield: 3 to 4 servings*

| | | | |
|---|---|---|---|
| Calories | 237 | Cholesterol | 0 mg |
| Fat | 2 g | Sodium | 567 mg |
| Saturated Fat | 0 g | Carbohydrate | 46 g |
| Mono | 0 g | Protein | 7 g |
| Poly | 0 g | | |

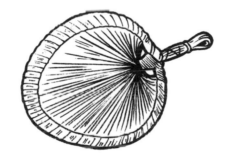

# VEGETABLES

CHINESE GREEN BEANS WITH PEANUTS

SICHUAN GREEN BEANS

STIR-FRIED GINGER BROCCOLI

GRILLED EGGPLANT WITH FILIPINO SALSA

ROASTED EGGPLANT WITH VIETNAMESE MINT SAUCE

SPICY EGGPLANT AND RED PEPPER, SICHUAN STYLE

CHINESE MARINATED MUSHROOMS

SPINACH AND MUSHROOMS, JAPANESE STYLE

JAPANESE GREEN PEPPERS WITH BONITO FLAKES (*Piman no Katsuo-Bushi Itame*)

STIR-FRIED TOFU WITH CHINESE CABBAGE AND RED PEPPER

JAPANESE STIR-FRIED TOFU, SCALLOPS, AND MIXED VEGETABLES

CHINESE FIVE-TREASURE VEGETABLE PLATTER

VIETNAMESE STIR-FRIED MIXED VEGETABLES WITH PEANUTS

INDONESIAN STIR-FRIED MIXED VEGETABLES (*Oseng-Oseng*)

SPICY THAI VEGETABLE MEDLEY

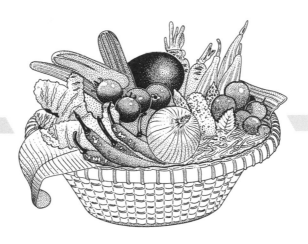

# Vegetables

FRESH VEGETABLES are harvested daily and stacked neatly in every stall in the markets of the Far East. This penchant for freshness extends to healthful preparations and presentations.

The natural flavors shine through in the Chinese Five-Treasure Vegetable Platter. Roasted Eggplant with Vietnamese Mint Sauce combines sweet, hot, and salty flavors with smoky roasted eggplant, topped with a refreshing mint sauce. Stir-frying heightens the subtle contrasts of ingredients in a Spicy Thai Vegetable Medley and the Japanese Stir-fried Tofu, Scallops, and Mixed Vegetables.

# CHINESE GREEN BEANS WITH PEANUTS

HERE IS an easily prepared Chinese green bean stir-fry that may be served hot or chilled.

3 tablespoons oyster-flavored sauce
3 tablespoons rice vinegar
1 teaspoon canola oil
2 teaspoons minced garlic
1 pound green beans, cut into 1½-inch lengths
2 to 3 tablespoons unsalted dry-roasted peanuts (optional)

In a small bowl, combine the oyster-flavored sauce and rice vinegar. Set aside.

Heat a nonstick skillet over medium heat. Add the oil and heat. Add the garlic and green beans. Stir-fry for about 3 minutes, or until seared on the outside. Add 3 tablespoons water. Reduce the heat to a simmer. Cover and cook, stirring occasionally, until crisp-tender, about 2 minutes. Add the sauce mixture. Toss together and cook until heated through, about 1 minute. Garnish with the peanuts, if using. Serve hot or refrigerate, covered, until chilled.

*Yield: 4 to 6 servings*

| | | | |
|---|---|---|---|
| Calories | 34 | Cholesterol | 2 mg |
| Fat | 1 g | Sodium | 287 mg |
| Saturated Fat | 0 g | Carbohydrate | 6 g |
| Mono | 0 g | Protein | 1 g |
| Poly | 0 g | | |

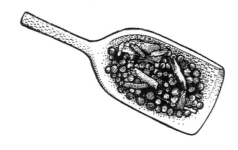

# SICHUAN GREEN BEANS

IN THIS typical Sichuan dish, the beans are brown and blistery on the outside but crisp and tender inside.

### Sauce Mixture
2 tablespoons vodka
$1^1/_2$ tablespoons low-sodium soy sauce
1 teaspoon hot chili oil

1 tablespoon canola oil
$1^1/_2$ pounds green beans, trimmed
$^1/_4$ pound lean ground pork (optional)
2 tablespoons Sichuan preserved mustard greens, rinsed with water to remove
    pepperiness, finely minced

Combine the sauce ingredients with 2 tablespoons water. Set aside.

Heat the oil in a nonstick skillet or stir-fry pan. Just before it begins to smoke, add the beans in batches. Stir-fry, tossing gently, until the beans are wrinkled and lightly browned. Remove each batch from the pan and set aside.

Add the pork, if using, and stir-fry, breaking it up until it begins to brown. Add the preserved mustard greens and stir for about 30 seconds. Add the beans and toss to combine. Add the sauce mixture and toss until the liquid is absorbed. Serve.

*Yield: 4 to 6 servings*

| | | | |
|---|---|---|---|
| Calories | 67 | Cholesterol | 0 mg |
| Fat | 4 g | Sodium | 145 mg |
| Saturated Fat | 0 g | Carbohydrate | 7 g |
| Mono | 2 g | Protein | 2 g |
| Poly | 1 g | | |

# STIR-FRIED GINGER BROCCOLI

THIS BROCCOLI dish is equally tasty served hot or at room temperature. It is both a refreshing summer dish and a warming winter stir-fry.

1½ pounds broccoli
1½ teaspoons canola oil
4 teaspoons peeled and finely shredded fresh ginger
Salt and freshly ground black pepper, to taste
1 tablespoon sesame seeds, toasted

Separate the broccoli into small florets. Peel the skin and cut the stems on the diagonal into 1¾ × ⅛-inch slices. Blanch the florets and stems for about 3 minutes, or until crisp-tender. Drain immediately and refresh under cold running water. Drain thoroughly.

Heat the oil in a large nonstick wok or skillet over medium heat. Add the ginger. Stir-fry until fragrant, about 20 seconds. Add the broccoli and stir-fry for 3 to 4 minutes, or until the broccoli is heated through. Season with salt and pepper. Add the sesame seeds and toss. Serve hot or chilled.

*Yield: 6 servings*

| | | | |
|---|---|---|---|
| Calories | 47 | Cholesterol | 0 mg |
| Fat | 2 g | Sodium | 25 mg |
| Saturated Fat | 0 g | Carbohydrate | 5 g |
| Mono | 1 g | Protein | 3 g |
| Poly | 1 g | | |

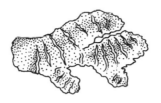

# GRILLED EGGPLANT WITH FILIPINO SALSA

FILIPINO CHEF Les Suniga, of the Princeville Resort on Kauai, taught this dish to me. He has modified the original dish from his native country by serving the eggplant sliced with the salsa on top. He says that at home, the eggplant would be stir-fried with the other ingredients and served cold as a salsa.

1 teaspoon olive oil
1/2 cup diced onion (1/4 inch)
1/2 cup diced tomatoes (1/4 inch)
1/2 cup chopped green onions
1 to 2 teaspoons fish sauce
Olive oil spray
3 to 4 small Japanese eggplants, cut lengthwise into 1/4-inch slices (about
    1 pound)
Salt and freshly ground black pepper, to taste

Heat the oil in a large nonstick skillet. Stir in the onion, tomatoes, and green onions. Cook until slightly soft, about 2 minutes. Sprinkle 1/2 teaspoon of the fish sauce on the mixture. Set the salsa aside.

Prepare a charcoal grill. When hot, spray the rack with the olive oil spray. Place the eggplant slices on the rack and grill on both sides until soft, about 3 minutes. Remove from the heat. Sprinkle the remaining fish sauce to taste on both sides of the eggplant.

To serve, place 2 eggplant slices in a V pattern on a serving plate. Place the salsa in the center. Season with salt and pepper. Serve hot as a vegetable side dish or at room temperature as an appetizer. If serving at room temperature, place the salsa on top of the eggplant when serving.

*Yield: 4 to 6 servings*

| | | | |
|---|---|---|---|
| Calories | 38 | Cholesterol | 0 mg |
| Fat | 1 g | Sodium | 43 mg |
| Saturated Fat | 0 g | Carbohydrate | 7 g |
| Mono | 1 g | Protein | 1 g |
| Poly | 0 g | | |

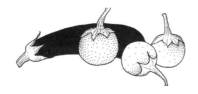

# ROASTED EGGPLANT WITH VIETNAMESE MINT SAUCE

SIMPLE ROASTED eggplant topped with a tangy sauce brightened with fresh mint can be served as a vegetable side dish for a main course or as an appetizer. You can roast the eggplant and make the sauce ahead if you like. When serving, just reheat the eggplant and add the sauce.

3 to 4 small Japanese eggplants (about 1 pound)
Canola oil spray
4 teaspoons fresh lime juice
4 teaspoons rice vinegar
4 teaspoons fish sauce
2 tablespoons plus 2 teaspoons sugar
3 cloves garlic, minced
1/4 cup finely chopped mint leaves
1/8 to 1/4 teaspoon red pepper powder (optional)
Dash of salt (optional)

Preheat the oven to 400 degrees.

Cut the eggplants on the diagonal into 3/4-inch slices. Lightly coat a baking sheet with canola oil spray. Place the eggplant slices side by side on the sheet. Lightly spray the top of the slices with more oil spray. Bake for 20 minutes, turn the slices over and bake for 10 minutes more, or until golden brown on each side.

While the eggplant is baking, combine the lime juice, rice vinegar, fish sauce, red pepper powder, sugar, garlic, mint, and salt, if using, in a small bowl. Stir until the sugar dissolves. Drizzle the sauce over the warm eggplant. Serve.

*Yield: 4 to 6 servings*

| | | | |
|---|---|---|---|
| Calories | 50 | Cholesterol | 0 mg |
| Fat | 0 g | Sodium | 156 mg |
| Saturated Fat | 0 g | Carbohydrate | 13 g |
| Mono | 0 g | Protein | 1 g |
| Poly | 0 g | | |

# SPICY EGGPLANT AND RED PEPPER, SICHUAN STYLE

THIS SPICE lover's dream comes from western Sichuan, China. Fiery chili paste with garlic, ginger, and more garlic will make your palate smolder. The dish is excellent served hot, room temperature, or cold. It will keep refrigerated for two to three days. The flavor will peak on about the second day. That's when I like to serve it, at room temperature, on toasted pita triangles or sesame crackers.

1 to 2 tablespoons Chinese chili paste with garlic, or to taste
1 tablespoon low-sodium soy sauce
1 tablespoon dry sherry
2 teaspoons red wine vinegar
2 teaspoons sugar
1 pound Japanese eggplants, trimmed
1 tablespoon plus 1 teaspoon canola oil
1 large red bell pepper, seeded and diced
1 tablespoon peeled and minced fresh ginger
1 tablespoon minced garlic
2 green onions, thinly sliced
Salt, to taste

In a small bowl, combine the chili paste, soy sauce, sherry, vinegar, and sugar. Set aside. Cut the eggplant into eighths lengthwise. Cut the strips into 1-inch pieces. Set aside.

Heat 1 teaspoon oil in a large nonstick skillet or stir-fry pan over medium heat. Add the bell pepper and stir-fry for 2 minutes, or until crisp-tender. Transfer to a plate. Set aside.

Heat 1 tablespoon oil in the skillet. Add the eggplant, ginger, and garlic. Stir-fry for 3 to 4 minutes, or until lightly browned. Add $^3/_4$ cup water. Reduce the heat to a simmer. Cover and simmer, stirring often, for about 5 minutes, or until the eggplant is tender. Stir in the bell pepper and half of the green onion.

Stir in the chili paste mixture. Stir for 1 to 2 minutes. Garnish with the remaining green onion. Serve hot, at room temperature, or cold.

*Yield: 4 to 6 servings*

| Calories | 77 | Cholesterol | 0 mg |
|---|---|---|---|
| Fat | 4 g | Sodium | 177 mg |
| Saturated Fat | 0 g | Carbohydrate | 11 g |
| Mono | 2 g | Protein | 2 g |
| Poly | 1 g | | |

# CHINESE MARINATED MUSHROOMS

BE SURE to purchase uniform-size white mushrooms that are tightly closed for this side dish, which may be served as an appetizer or as an accompaniment to any meal. Make it the day before you plan to serve it.

$^1/_2$ pound small white button mushrooms, cleaned and trimmed
1 clove garlic, minced
$^1/_2$ cup minced onion
$^1/_4$ teaspoon red pepper flakes
1 tablespoon sugar
2 tablespoons low-sodium soy sauce
1 tablespoon vodka
2 tablespoons balsamic vinegar
3 tablespoons fat-free low-sodium Chicken Stock (page 60) or water
Salt and freshly ground pepper, to taste

Place the mushrooms in a bowl.

Combine the garlic, onion, red pepper flakes, sugar, soy sauce, vodka, vinegar, and stock in a small pan. Bring to a boil, stirring until the sugar dissolves. Pour the boiling mixture over the mushrooms and toss well to combine. Refrigerate, covered, tossing occasionally, for 1 day. Season with salt and pepper. Drain and serve.

*Yield: 6 to 8 servings*

| | | | |
|---|---|---|---|
| Calories | 29 | Cholesterol | 0 mg |
| Fat | 0 g | Sodium | 141 mg |
| Saturated Fat | 0 g | Carbohydrate | 5 g |
| Mono | 0 g | Protein | 1 g |
| Poly | 0 g | | |

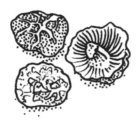

# SPINACH AND MUSHROOMS, JAPANESE STYLE

HERE IS an easily prepared dish from my Japanese friends Sumie Ishikawa.

1 pound fresh spinach, washed, stems removed, cut into 1-inch pieces
6 Chinese dried black mushrooms, soaked in warm water for 20 minutes, stems
    removed, caps sliced
2 tablespoons sake
1 tablespoon sugar
1 1/2 tablespoons low-sodium soy sauce
1 egg, lightly beaten

Boil 1/2 cup water in a wok. Add the spinach and stir until wilted. Add the mushrooms and stir for 30 seconds. Add the sake, sugar, and soy sauce. Toss to combine.

Add the egg in the center of the spinach. Do not stir. Cover for 30 seconds to 1 minute, or until the egg sets. Remove from heat. Slide onto a serving dish. Serve immediately.

*Yield: 4 servings*

| | | | |
|---|---|---|---|
| Calories | 78 | Cholesterol | 53 mg |
| Fat | 2 g | Sodium | 276 mg |
| Saturated Fat | 0 g | Carbohydrate | 11 g |
| Mono | 1 g | Protein | 6 g |
| Poly | 0 g | | |

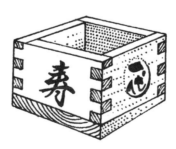

# JAPANESE GREEN PEPPERS WITH BONITO FLAKES

## PIMAN NO KATSUO-BUSHI ITAME

CRUNCHY GREEN peppers and smoky dried bonito flakes produce this intriguing side dish introduced to me by Sumie Ishikawa, who is from Yokohama.

2 teaspoons canola oil
2 green bell peppers, cut into julienne
1/3 cup (loosely packed) dried shaved bonito flakes
1 to 2 teaspoons low-sodium soy sauce

Heat the oil in a medium nonstick skillet over medium heat. Add the peppers and sauté until crisp. Add the bonito flakes and soy sauce to taste. Stir for 30 seconds. Serve.

*Yield: 4 servings*

| | | | |
|---|---|---|---|
| Calories | 48 | Cholesterol | 9 mg |
| Fat | 2 g | Sodium | 71 mg |
| Saturated Fat | 0 g | Carbohydrate | 2 g |
| Mono | 1 g | Protein | 4 g |
| Poly | 0 g | | |

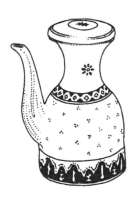

# STIR-FRIED TOFU WITH CHINESE CABBAGE AND RED PEPPER

THE NUTRITIONAL simplicity of Chinese food shines through in this dish. It is my version of a stir-fry created for me by specialist chef Lilay Layaoen of the Princeville Resort on Kauai. She says this was her favorite Chinese dish when she lived in the Philippines.

*Sauce Mixture*
1/2 to 1 1/2 teaspoons red pepper flakes
3 tablespoons oyster-flavored sauce
2 tablespoons low-sodium soy sauce
1 tablespoon sugar

2 teaspoons canola oil
1 tablespoon peeled and minced ginger
2 tablespoons minced garlic
1 red bell pepper, cut into 1-inch pieces
3/4 pound Chinese or napa cabbage, trimmed, leaves cut into 2-inch pieces
1 cake (14 ounces) firm tofu, drained and cut into 1/2-inch cubes
2 cups fresh bean sprouts
2 green onions, cut on the diagonal into 2-inch pieces
2 teaspoons cornstarch dissolved in 4 teaspoons cold water
Salt and freshly ground black pepper, to taste

Combine the red pepper flakes, oyster-flavored sauce, soy sauce, and sugar in a small dish. Stir and set aside.

Heat the oil in nonstick wok or large skillet over medium heat. Add the ginger, garlic, and red bell pepper. Stir-fry for 2 minutes, or until the pepper is almost crisp-tender. Add the cabbage. Stir-fry until the cabbage is almost wilted. Add the tofu, bean sprouts, green onions, and oyster-flavored sauce mixture. Toss gently for 1 minute until heated through and the cabbage is wilted. Recombine the sauce mixture and add to the pan. Cook, stirring gently, until the sauce is shiny. Season with salt and pepper. Serve.

*Yield: 4 to 6 servings*

| | | | |
|---|---|---|---|
| Calories | 170 | Cholesterol | 2 mg |
| Fat | 8 g | Sodium | 475 mg |
| Saturated Fat | 1 g | Carbohydrate | 15 g |
| Mono | 2 g | Protein | 14 g |
| Poly | 4 g | | |

# JAPANESE STIR-FRIED TOFU, SCALLOPS, AND MIXED VEGETABLES

THIS SIMPLE, nutritious tofu combination is a favorite in the home of Sumie Ishikawa, who successfully made the transition from Yokohama, Japan, to Schaumburg, Illinois.

1 package (2 ounces) bean threads
2 teaspoons canola oil
4 teaspoons peeled and minced ginger
3 stalks celery, thinly sliced on the diagonal
6 Chinese dried black mushrooms, soaked in warm water for 20 minutes, stems removed, caps coarsely chopped
16 bay scallops (about 8 ounces)
1 cake (14 ounces) firm tofu, drained and cut into 1/2-inch cubes
2 tablespoons low-sodium soy sauce
1 tablespoon sake
1 tablespoon cornstarch dissolved in 2 tablespoons water

Heat 4 quarts of water to a boil. Add the bean threads and stir to separate. When the water returns to a boil, stir again to separate. Cook until translucent, about 30 seconds. (Do not overcook.) Drain. Refresh with cold water. Drain for 5 minutes, lifting occasionally to help the noodles to dry. Cut into 2-inch lengths with kitchen shears.

Heat the oil in a nonstick skillet over medium heat. Add the ginger and stir until fragrant, about 20 seconds. Add the celery and mushrooms and stir for 30 seconds. Add the bean threads and stir for 30 seconds. Add the scallops and stir for about 3 minutes, or until the scallops start to turn opaque. Add the tofu and cook until heated. Gently stir in the soy sauce and sake. Recombine the cornstarch mixture and stir into the pan. Cook until shiny. Serve immediately.

*Yield: 4 to 6 servings*

| | | | |
|---|---|---|---|
| Calories | 198 | Cholesterol | 16 mg |
| Fat | 8 g | Sodium | 285 mg |
| Saturated Fat | 1 g | Carbohydrate | 15 g |
| Mono | 2 g | Protein | 19 g |
| Poly | 4 g | | |

# CHINESE FIVE-TREASURE VEGETABLE PLATTER

A RAINBOW of colors faces you in this lightly sauced banquet dish from Beijing. Use your own creativity by choosing vegetables of your own choice instead of my suggestions. Be sure to choose vegetables in complementary colors to arrange in a decorative pattern on a platter.

I like to serve the vegetables at room temperature. That gives me plenty of time to arrange the food presentation. Then I reheat the sauce and pour it over the vegetables at serving time. This recipe may easily be doubled.

> 1 pound asparagus, tough ends removed and stems peeled
> 1 pound baby carrots, trimmed
> 1 can (15 ounces) straw mushrooms, drained
> 1 can (15 ounces) baby corn, drained
> 2 cups fat-free low-sodium Chicken Stock (page 60)
> 1 tablespoon dry sherry
> 1 tablespoon low-sodium soy sauce
> 1 teaspoon sugar
> 3 medium tomatoes, peeled, quartered, and seeded
> 2 tablespoons cornstarch dissolved in 1/4 cup cold water
> 1/2 teaspoon Asian sesame oil

Separately blanch the asparagus and carrots in boiling water until barely tender. Drain. Set aside. Refresh under cold water. Separately blanch the mushrooms and corn in boiling water for about 15 seconds. Drain. Refresh under cold water. Set aside.

Combine the stock, sherry, soy sauce, and sugar in a 2-quart saucepan. Reheat the mushrooms in the mixture. Drain, reserving the mixture. Place in the center of a round platter. Reheat the corn, carrots, asparagus, and tomatoes, one by one in the mixture, always reserving the mixture. Place the vegetables in groups in a pinwheel design around the edge of the mushrooms.

Bring the mixture to a boil. Recombine the cornstarch mixture. Add to the saucepan and stir until translucent and thickened. Add the sesame oil. Stir. Pour the sauce mixture over the vegetables.

*Yield: 8 servings*

| | | | |
|---|---|---|---|
| Calories | 124 | Cholesterol | 0 mg |
| Fat | 2 g | Sodium | 350 mg |
| Saturated Fat | 0 g | Carbohydrate | 24 g |
| Mono | 0 g | Protein | 6 g |
| Poly | 1 g | | |

# VIETNAMESE STIR-FRIED MIXED VEGETABLES WITH PEANUTS

A SPARKLING combination of vegetables is found in this Vietnamese stir-fry. Make your own choice of vegetables if you like, but be sure to cut them the same size and stir-fry the longer-cooking vegetables first.

2 teaspoons canola oil
1 tablespoon peeled and minced fresh ginger
2 medium carrots, julienned
3 stalks celery, cut on the diagonal into 1/4-inch slices
1 red bell pepper, cut into 1/4-inch julienne
1 green bell pepper, cut into 1/4-inch julienne
4 ounces mushrooms, cleaned and sliced
3 green onions, sliced on the diagonal into 2-inch pieces
2 tablespoons fat-free low-sodium Chicken Stock (page 60) or water
2 teaspoons fish sauce
Freshly ground black pepper, to taste
1 tablespoon chopped fresh coriander (cilantro) (optional)
1/4 cup unsalted dry-roasted peanuts, coarsely chopped (optional)

Heat the oil in a nonstick stir-fry pan or skillet over medium heat until hot. Add the ginger, carrots, and celery and stir fry for 1 minute. Add the red and green bell peppers, mushrooms, and green onions. Stir until the vegetables just begin to soften. Stir in the stock, fish sauce, and black pepper. Garnish with fresh coriander and peanuts, if using. Serve immediately.

*Yield: 4 servings*

| | | | |
|---|---|---|---|
| Calories | 78 | Cholesterol | 0 mg |
| Fat | 3 g | Sodium | 166 mg |
| Saturated Fat | 0 g | Carbohydrate | 13 g |
| Mono | 1 g | Protein | 3 g |
| Poly | 1 g | | |

# INDONESIAN STIR-FRIED MIXED VEGETABLES

## OSENG-OSENG

THE NATURAL flavors of vegetables are heightened by chilies in this dish taught to me by Joelina Soejono, wife of Soejono Soerjoatmodjo, Consul General of Indonesia in Chicago.

If galangal is unavailable, she substitutes ginger.

1/2 cup thinly sliced onion
2 shallots, thinly sliced
2 cloves garlic, thinly sliced
2 quarter-size pieces peeled galangal, crushed
1 bay leaf
3 small carrots, thinly sliced on the diagonal
3/4 pound green beans, trimmed and cut on the diagonal into 1 1/2-inch lengths
1 red bell pepper, seeded and julienned
3/4 cup baby corn, cut in half lengthwise
2 red chilies, seeds removed and thinly sliced
1 green chili, seeds removed and thinly sliced
1 tablespoon oyster-flavored sauce
Salt, to taste

Heat the oil in a nonstick stir-fry pan or large nonstick skillet. Add the onion, shallots, garlic, galangal, and bay leaf. Stir until the onion is translucent. Add the carrots, green beans, and bell pepper, and stir for 1 to 2 minutes. Add the corn and stir for 30 seconds. Add the red and green chilies and oyster-flavored sauce. Stir for 30 seconds. Season with salt. The vegetables should be crunchy.

*Yield: 4 to 6 servings*

| | | | |
|---|---|---|---|
| Calories | 136 | Cholesterol | 1 mg |
| Fat | 1 g | Sodium | 116 mg |
| Saturated Fat | 0 g | Carbohydrate | 28 g |
| Mono | 0 g | Protein | 4 g |
| Poly | 0 g | | |

# SPICY THAI VEGETABLE MEDLEY

IN THIS easy stir-fry, hot chilies and mint add zip to a colorful bouquet of eggplant, zucchini, red pepper, and straw mushrooms. Button mushrooms and fresh coriander may be substituted for the straw mushrooms and mint.

1 teaspoon olive oil
1 shallot, thinly sliced
1 teaspoon peeled and minced fresh ginger
1 teaspoon minced garlic
1 to 2 red chilies, seeded and minced
1/2 pound Japanese eggplant, cut into 1/4-inch dice
1 large red bell pepper, cut into 1/4-inch dice
1/2 pound zucchini, cut into 1/4-inch dice
1 can (8 ounces) straw mushrooms, drained (optional)
2 teaspoons fish sauce
2 teaspoons low-sodium soy sauce
1/2 cup mint leaves
Sprigs of mint, for garnish

Heat the oil in a large nonstick skillet over medium heat. Add the shallot, ginger, garlic, and chilies and stir-fry until the shallot is translucent, 20 seconds. Add the eggplant and bell pepper. Stir-fry for 4 to 6 minutes, or until the eggplant is almost tender. Add the zucchini and straw mushrooms. Stir-fry for 1 to 2 minutes, or until the vegetables are tender. Stir in the fish and soy sauce. Remove the pan from the heat. Add the mint leaves and stir until wilted. Serve garnished with mint sprigs.

*Yield: 6 servings*

| | | | |
|---|---|---|---|
| Calories | 44 | Cholesterol | 0 mg |
| Fat | 1 g | Sodium | 138 mg |
| Saturated Fat | 0 g | Carbohydrate | 8 g |
| Mono | 1 g | Protein | 2 g |
| Poly | 0 g | | |

# SALADS

Japanese Vegetable Salad with Sesame-Miso Dressing

Indonesian Mixed Vegetable Salad with Peanut Dressing (*Gado Gado*)

Tomatoes Stuffed with Spiced Eggplant

Thai Spiced Fruit Salad (*Yam Polami*)

Jicama, Carrot, Red Pepper, and Mesclun Salad with Lime Dressing

Indonesian Spicy Fruit Salad (*Rujak*)

Mango Salad

Green Papaya Salad

Chicken Salad with Papaya Seed and Orange-Ginger Dressing

Vietnamese Chicken Salad

Hot-and-Sour Seafood Salad

Tomatoes Stuffed with Spicy Chicken Salad

Vietnamese Shrimp Salad

Basmati Rice and Vegetable Salad

Japanese Smoked Salmon Salad

Thai Noodle and Vegetable Salad

Soba Noodle Salad

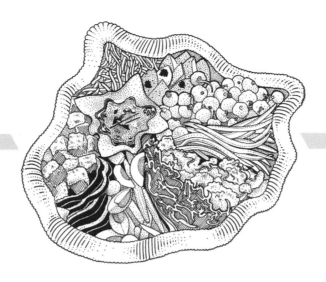

# SALADS

THE COMPLEX flavors of the Pacific Rim are combined in freshly prepared and colorfully presented salads to create a touch of excitement in a meal, whether they are served as a first course, side dish, or light entree. The selection in this chapter highlights classics from Vietnam, Japan, Indonesia, and Thailand, as well as my own interpretations of Pacific Rim salads. You'll find salads made from vegetables, fruit, chicken, seafood, rice, and noodles.

Consider serving a meal of many small salads to provide a sampling of seasonings, color, texture, and lingering flavors. I recommend including the Indonesian *Gado Gado*, a Thai Spiced Fruit Salad, and Mango Salad—or use your own imagination. Tomatoes Stuffed with Spicy Chicken Salad or Tomatoes Stuffed with Spiced Eggplant work equally well as a first course or as a side dish.

One of my favorite luncheon salads is Hawaiian Chicken Salad with Papaya Seed and Orange-Ginger Dressing. For a buffet or potluck I like the Hot-and-Sour Seafood Salad or Basmati Rice and Vegetable Salad.

# JAPANESE VEGETABLE SALAD WITH SESAME-MISO DRESSING

THIS AROMATIC tangy sesame and miso dressing transforms ordinary vegetables into an unusual salad.

**Sesame-Miso Dressing**
2 to 3 tablespoons sesame seeds, toasted
2 to 3 tablespoons white miso
$1/3$ cup *Dashi* (page 61)
2 tablespoons low-sodium soy sauce
2 teaspoons prepared mustard
$1^1/2$ tablespoons rice vinegar
1 tablespoon canola oil

2 carrots, cut into 2-inch-long julienne
1 cucumber, seeded and cut into 2-inch-long julienne
4 ounces snow peas, string removed, blanched, and cut on the diagonal into julienne
1 red bell pepper, seeded and cut into 2-inch-long julienne
4 ounces daikon, peeled and cut into 2-inch-long julienne
Romaine or Boston lettuce leaves

To prepare the dressing, process the sesame seeds to a paste in a blender or mini food processor. Place the miso in a small bowl, add the dashi, and stir to dissolve the miso. Add the soy sauce, mustard, vinegar, and oil. Stir to combine. Set aside for 30 minutes.

Arrange the vegetables on the lettuce leaves. Serve the dressing separately, allowing your guests to serve themselves.

*Yield: 4 to 6 servings*

| | | | |
|---|---|---|---|
| Calories | 95 | Cholesterol | 0 mg |
| Fat | 5 g | Sodium | 420 mg |
| Saturated Fat | 0 g | Carbohydrate | 12 g |
| Mono | 2 g | Protein | 4 g |
| Poly | 2 g | | |

# INDONESIAN MIXED VEGETABLE SALAD WITH PEANUT DRESSING

## GADO GADO

*GADO GADO,* one of Indonesia's classic vegetable salads, is dressed in a creamy peanut sauce. Its presentation is of great importance. It should be served on a large platter with careful attention to the decorative arrangement of the vegetables. It is perfect for a luncheon, light supper, or buffet table.

The peanut dressing tastes better when prepared a day ahead. If the dressing becomes too thick, add evaporated skim milk or water to thin it to the desired consistency. Since the vegetables should be prepared ahead and cooled to room temperature before serving, this is the ultimate dish for entertaining.

Coconut milk is used in Indonesia for the preparation of the dressing. I have substituted evaporated skim milk and coconut flavoring. If you wish to use coconut milk, substitute one cup medium coconut milk for the evaporated milk.

2 medium potatoes, scrubbed
2 medium carrots, thinly sliced
3 ounces green beans, trimmed and cut into 2-inch lengths
4 ounces fresh bean sprouts, washed and drained
2 cups shredded cabbage

**Peanut Dressing**
1 teaspoon canola oil
$1/2$ teaspoon peeled and minced fresh ginger
1 clove garlic, finely chopped
2 tablespoons finely chopped onion
1 red chili, seeded and finely chopped
$3/4$ cup evaporated skim milk
1 teaspoon brown sugar, or to taste
$1/3$ cup plus 2 tablespoons reduced-fat peanut butter
$1/8$ teaspoon coconut flavoring
Fresh lime juice, to taste
Salt, to taste

**Garnish**

$\frac{1}{2}$ small cucumber, cut in half, seeded, and sliced
Sprigs of watercress (optional)

Boil the potatoes, peel, and thinly slice. In a large saucepan of boiling water, blanch the carrots and green beans separately for 2 minutes. Drain. Refresh with cold water. Drain. Set aside. Blanch the bean sprouts and cabbage separately in boiling water for 20 seconds. Rinse under cold water. Drain well. Set aside.

To make the dressing, heat the oil in a nonstick saucepan over medium heat. Add the ginger, garlic, and onion. Cook until the onion is translucent, about 2 minutes. Add the chili, evaporated skim milk, $\frac{1}{4}$ cup water, brown sugar, and peanut butter. Whisk to blend the mixture. Bring to a boil. Reduce the heat and simmer, stirring occasionally, until the sauce has thickened, but is still thin enough to pour, 3 to 4 minutes. If the sauce becomes too thick, whisk in more evaporated skim milk or water. Add the coconut flavoring, lime juice, and salt. Set aside. Reheat when serving.

Arrange the vegetables in separate sections on a large platter in a decorative pattern. Surround the platter with slices of cucumber. Pour the peanut sauce over the salad. Garnish with watercress, if desired. Serve at room temperature.

*Yield: 8 to 10 servings*

| | | | |
|---|---|---|---|
| Calories | 81 | Cholesterol | 1 mg |
| Fat | 2 g | Sodium | 53 mg |
| Saturated Fat | 0 g | Carbohydrate | 13 g |
| Mono | 1 g | Protein | 4 g |
| Poly | 1 g | | |

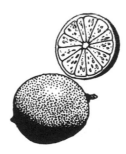

# TOMATOES STUFFED WITH SPICED EGGPLANT

THIS IS my rendition of an elegant dish I tasted at the luxurious Manele Bay Hotel on Lana'i, where Philippe Padovani presides as Executive Chef. Ripe tomatoes filled to the brim with roasted eggplant and diced tomatoes are served on a bed of mesclun. You may substitute half a cup of chopped fresh basil for the mint. Instead of stuffing the tomatoes, Chef Padovani tops carefully molded ovals of the eggplant salad with a carved tomato petal.

4 medium, firm, ripe tomatoes
Salt
1 clove garlic, crushed
1 Italian eggplant (about 1 pound)
Olive oil spray
2 teaspoons Dijon mustard
1 teaspoon sherry wine vinegar
1 tablespoon plus 1 teaspoon extra virgin olive oil
$^1/_2$ cup finely minced onion
$^1/_2$ teaspoon finely minced garlic
$1^1/_2$ cups diced tomatoes, including pulp from tomato shells
$^1/_4$ cup mint leaves, minced
Freshly ground black pepper, to taste
Whole mint leaves, for garnish
Mesclun or lettuce leaves

Cut a thin slice off the stem end of each tomato. Scoop out the pulp and reserve it. Season the tomato shells lightly with salt and rub the inside with a garlic clove. Invert on a rack to drain for about 15 minutes. Dry the inside of the tomatoes with a paper towel.

Preheat the oven to 375 degrees.

Cut the eggplant lengthwise in half and score in a $1^1/_2$-inch diamond pattern. Line a baking sheet with foil. Spray the foil lightly with oil. Place the eggplant, cut side up, on the baking sheet and bake in the middle of the oven until very soft, 30 to 35 minutes. Cool slightly. Scoop out the flesh with a large spoon and discard the shells. Finely chop the pulp.

Meanwhile, stir together the mustard, vinegar, and 1 tablespoon oil in a bowl until blended. Set aside.

Heat remaining 1 teaspoon oil in a nonstick skillet over medium heat. Add the onion and garlic and cook until the onion is translucent, about 2 minutes. Add the eggplant and tomatoes. Cook until the tomatoes are soft and the liquid is absorbed, about 3 to 4 minutes. Add the minced mint and stir until wilted. Remove from the heat. Add the mustard mixture and season with salt and pepper.

Fill the tomatoes with the eggplant-tomato mixture. Garnish with mint leaves. Serve on a bed of mesclun.

*Yield: 4 servings*

| | | | |
|---|---|---|---|
| Calories | 115 | Cholesterol | 0 mg |
| Fat | 5 g | Sodium | 57 mg |
| Saturated Fat | 1 g | Carbohydrate | 19 g |
| Mono | 3 g | Protein | 3 g |
| Poly | 1 g | | |

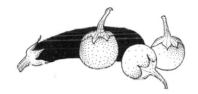

# THAI SPICED FRUIT SALAD

## YAM POLAMI

THIS SALAD would be served as an afternoon snack or as a vivid contrast during a meal in Thailand. It is best when made from underripe fruits; it is often combined with cooked shrimp. For an unusual presentation, serve it in orange shells.

⅓ cup fresh lime juice
1 small green apple, such as Granny Smith, peeled, cored, cut into quarters, and
    thinly sliced
1 underripe pear, peeled, cored, cut into quarters, and thinly sliced
Vegetable oil spray
3 cloves garlic, thinly sliced
1 large shallot, thinly sliced
Salt, to taste
½ cup red seedless grapes, halved
1 orange or tangerine, peeled and sectioned
½ grapefruit, peeled and sectioned
1 firm papaya or mango, peeled, cut in half, seeded, and thinly sliced
2 to 3 teaspoons brown sugar, or to taste

### Garnish
2 tablespoons chopped unsalted dry-roasted peanuts
Mint leaves
1 or 2 red chilies, seeded and thinly sliced (optional)

Pour a little of the lime juice on the sliced apple and pear to prevent discoloration.

Preheat the oven to 400 degrees. Spray a nonstick baking sheet lightly with oil.

Sprinkle the garlic and shallot slices over the baking sheet to separate them. Spray oil evenly over the shallot. Bake in the center of the oven, stirring occasionally, for about 15 minutes, or until brown and crisp. Season with salt, if desired. Let cool completely.

Combine the fruits in a bowl. Combine sugar, salt, and the remaining lime juice. Stir. Pour over the fruits. Garnish with peanuts, mint, and chili, if using. Serve chilled or at room temperature.

| Calories | 171 | Cholesterol | 0 mg |
|---|---|---|---|
| Fat | 3 g | Sodium | 9 mg |
| Saturated Fat | 0 g | Carbohydrate | 38 g |
| Mono | 2 g | Protein | 2 g |
| Poly | 0 g | | |

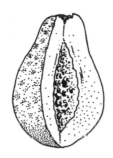

# JICAMA, CARROT, RED PEPPER, AND MESCLUN SALAD WITH LIME DRESSING

HAWAIIAN COLORS shine in this sparkling combination of crisp white jicama, carrots, and red peppers topped with a tart lime dressing.

### Lime Dressing
1/4 cup fresh lime juice
1 teaspoon peeled and minced fresh ginger
2 teaspoons extra virgin olive oil
Salt and freshly ground black pepper, to taste

2 cups peeled and julienned jicama
1 medium red bell pepper, seeded and julienned
1 medium carrot, julienned
1/4 cup finely chopped red onion
3 ounces mesclun or other mixed salad greens
4 radicchio leaves
4 sprigs of mint, leaves only

To prepare the dressing, combine the lime juice and ginger in a bowl. Whisk in the oil until blended. Season with salt and pepper. Set aside.

Toss the jicama, bell pepper, carrot, red onion, and dressing in a bowl. Arrange the mesclun around the edge of each plate. Place a radicchio leaf in the center. Spoon the jicama mixture on top of the radicchio leaf. Garnish with mint leaves and serve.

*Yield: 4 servings*

| | | | |
|---|---|---|---|
| Calories | 95 | Cholesterol | 0 mg |
| Fat | 3 g | Sodium | 11 mg |
| Saturated Fat | 0 g | Carbohydrate | 17 g |
| Mono | 2 g | Protein | 3 g |
| Poly | 0 g | | |

# INDONESIAN SPICY FRUIT SALAD

## RUJAK

*RUJAK* IS an example of the Javanese penchant for combining hot, sweet, and tangy flavors. They prefer to use fruit that is not fully ripe to produce the best combination of sharp and sour tastes. Serve the salad as a light meal or as part of a larger meal with savory dishes. The dressing can also be served in individual bowls for dipping. The dressing tastes better when made a day ahead to allow flavors to blend.

1 firm green apple, such as Granny Smith, peeled, cored, quartered, and cut into
$1/4$-inch slices
1 grapefruit, peeled and sectioned
1 small orange, peeled and sectioned
1 firm mango or slightly underripe pear, peeled and cut into bite-size pieces
$1/2$ fresh pineapple, peeled and cut into $1/2$-inch wedges
$1/2$ cucumber, peeled, halved, seeded, and cut into thin slices

*Dressing*
1 red chili, seeded and finely chopped
1 to 2 tablespoons dark brown sugar, or to taste
1 tablespoon low-sodium soy sauce
1 teaspoon tamarind pulp dissolved in 4 tablespoons hot water or 1 tablespoon
fresh lime juice plus 3 tablespoons water

Combine the fruits and cucumber in a serving bowl. Combine the dressing ingredients in a small bowl and stir to mix. Pour the dressing over the salad. Toss to combine. Serve at room temperature.

*Yield: 6 servings*

| | | | |
|---|---|---|---|
| Calories | 112 | Cholesterol | 0 mg |
| Fat | 1 g | Sodium | 91 mg |
| Saturated Fat | 0 g | Carbohydrate | 28 g |
| Mono | 0 g | Protein | 1 g |
| Poly | 0 g | | |

# MANGO SALAD

WHEN AROMATIC ripe mangoes are in season, this refreshing salad from southern India is one of my favorite summer dishes. Ripe peaches can be substituted.

1 to 2 large ripe mangoes (about 2 pounds)
1/3 cup plain non-fat yogurt
1/2 teaspoon coconut flavoring
1 to 2 green chilies, seeded and finely shredded
1 teaspoon peeled and minced fresh ginger
2 tablespoons finely chopped mint leaves
1/8 teaspoon freshly grated nutmeg
2 teaspoons fresh lime juice
1 teaspoon honey, or to taste
Salt and freshly ground black pepper, to taste

Peel the mangoes and cut the flesh into 1/2-inch cubes.

Whisk the yogurt with a fork until smooth and creamy. Combine the coconut flavoring, chilies, ginger, mint, nutmeg, lime juice, and honey in a bowl and stir. Add the mangoes and gently stir to combine. Season with salt and pepper. Check for sweetness. If the mangoes are not fully ripe, add more honey to taste. Stir to combine. Serve chilled or at room temperature.

*Yield: 4 to 6 servings*

| | | | |
|---|---|---|---|
| Calories | 114 | Cholesterol | 0 mg |
| Fat | 0 g | Sodium | 51 mg |
| Saturated Fat | 0 g | Carbohydrate | 28 g |
| Mono | 0 g | Protein | 2 g |
| Poly | 0 g | | |

# GREEN PAPAYA SALAD

IN THE Philippines and in Southeast Asia, this salad is made with green (unripe) papaya, which is available in Asian grocery stores in the United States. A good substitute is Granny Smith apples. Lilay Layaoen, specialist chef of the Princeville Resort on Kauai, says the salad should be tart and sweet with a bite of chili.

2 green papayas, peeled, seeded, and cut into $1\frac{1}{2}$-inch-long julienne (about 3 cups)
$\frac{3}{4}$ cup chopped ripe tomatoes
$\frac{1}{2}$ pound medium shrimp, cooked
1 to 2 green chilies, seeded and chopped
2 green onions, finely sliced
2 teaspoons fresh lime juice
$\frac{1}{3}$ cup (lightly packed) light brown sugar, or to taste
2 tablespoons fish sauce, or to taste
2 to 3 tablespoons coarsely chopped unsalted dry-roasted peanuts

Toss the papaya, tomatoes, shrimp, chilies, and green onions in a bowl. Combine the lime juice, brown sugar, and fish sauce and pour over the salad. Refrigerate for 1 hour. Serve garnished with peanuts.

*Yield: about 6 cups*

| | | | |
|---|---|---|---|
| Calories | 26 | Cholesterol | 9 mg |
| Fat | 0 g | Sodium | 40 mg |
| Saturated Fat | 0 g | Carbohydrate | 3 g |
| Mono | 0 g | Protein | 1 g |
| Poly | 0 g | | |

# CHICKEN SALAD WITH PAPAYA SEED AND ORANGE-GINGER DRESSING

WHET YOUR guests' appetites with this colorful salad full of Asian flavors: ginger, garlic, lemon grass, lime juice, soy sauce, and peppery papaya seeds. This salad was inspired by Daniel Delbrel, Executive Chef at the Princeville Resort on Kauai. The salad components may be prepared ahead and assembled just before serving.

### *Sauce Mixture*
2 tablespoons low-sodium soy sauce
1 tablespoon sugar
2 cloves garlic, minced
1 quarter-size slice of peeled fresh ginger
1 stalk lemon grass, bottom 6 inches only, minced
1 green onion, minced
2 tablespoons fresh lime juice

### *Dressing*
1/3 teaspoon coarsely chopped shallots
1/2 teaspoon rinsed papaya seeds, crushed
1/2 teaspoon peeled and coarsely chopped fresh ginger
1/2 teaspoon Dijon mustard
1/3 cup fresh orange juice
1 tablespoon extra virgin olive oil
1/2 teaspoon Asian sesame oil
Salt, to taste

1 teaspoon canola oil
1 1/2 pounds boneless and skinless chicken breasts, julienned
1 medium red bell pepper, seeded and julienned
6 ounces mesclun greens
1 ripe papaya, peeled, seeded, and julienned
1 teaspoon sesame seeds, toasted (optional)

Combine the sauce ingredients and 1 tablespoon water in a bowl. Set aside.

In a blender, puree the shallots, ginger, papaya seeds, mustard, and orange juice. Add 2 tablespoons water and the olive and sesame oils and blend until emulsified. Season with salt. Chill for at least 1 hour before serving.

Heat the canola oil in a nonstick skillet. Add the chicken and stir-fry for 1 minute. Add the bell pepper. Stir-fry until crisp-tender, about 2 minutes. Add the sauce mixture and stir for about 30 seconds. Remove and set aside.

Place the mesclun on individual serving plates. Drizzle the dressing over the mesclun. Arrange the cooked chicken mixture on top. Garnish with papaya. Sprinkle with sesame seeds. Serve immediately.

*Yield: 4 to 6 servings*

| Calories | 206 | Cholesterol | 49 mg |
|---|---|---|---|
| Fat | 6 g | Sodium | 232 mg |
| Saturated Fat | 1 g | Carbohydrate | 19 g |
| Mono | 3 g | Protein | 20 g |
| Poly | 1 g | | |

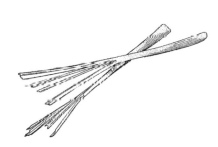

# VIETNAMESE CHICKEN SALAD

COLORFUL VEGETABLES and chicken are dressed with a sweet-and-sour spicy sauce. Cool and refreshing, this salad is irresistible.

2 cups fat-free low-sodium Chicken Stock (page 60)
1½ pounds boneless and skinless chicken breasts
1 cup fresh bean sprouts
2 cloves garlic, finely chopped
1 to 2 red chilies, seeded, finely julienned
3 tablespoons fresh lime juice
2 tablespoons fish sauce
2 tablespoons rice vinegar
2 teaspoons sugar
1 large carrot, cut into 1½-inch-long julienne
1 medium cucumber, peeled, seeded, and cut into 1½-inch-long julienne
1 medium red onion, very thinly sliced
⅓ cup chopped fresh coriander (cilantro) or mint leaves
6 romaine lettuce leaves

### Garnish
Whole coriander (cilantro) or mint leaves
2 to 3 tablespoons unsalted dry-roasted peanuts, chopped (optional)

Bring the stock to a boil in a large saucepan. Add the chicken breasts. Bring back to a full boil. Reduce the heat to low, cover, and simmer for about 15 minutes, or until the chicken is no longer pink. Remove the chicken from the liquid and let cool. Discard the skin. Shred the chicken into 2-inch-long pieces.

Blanch the bean sprouts in boiling water for 30 to 40 seconds. Drain. Refresh with cold water. Drain.

Mix the garlic, chilies, lime juice, fish sauce, vinegar, and sugar in a small bowl. Stir until the sugar is dissolved. Set aside.

Combine the chicken, bean sprouts, carrot, cucumber, red onion, and fresh coriander in a large bowl. Add the dressing mixture and toss to mix well. Arrange lettuce leaves on a serving platter. Place the salad on the lettuce leaves. Sprinkle fresh coriander and peanuts, if using, on top of the salad.

| Calories | 188 | Cholesterol | 69 mg |
|---|---|---|---|
| Fat | 3 g | Sodium | 410 mg |
| Saturated Fat | 1 g | Carbohydrate | 10 g |
| Mono | 1 g | Protein | 29 g |
| Poly | 1 g | | |

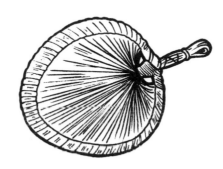

# HOT-AND-SOUR SEAFOOD SALAD

IN THIS colorful Chinese salad shrimps, scallops, red bell peppers, and cucumbers are combined with a hot-and-sour sauce. It makes an attractive presentation on a buffet table. You may prepare the ingredients and sauce ahead and add the sauce when ready to serve.

*Sauce Mixture*
2 tablespoons canola oil
2 to 4 dried red chilies
1 teaspoon five-spice powder
1/4 cup fat-free low-sodium Chicken Stock (page 60)
1 teaspoon low-sodium soy sauce
2 tablespoons red wine vinegar
2 tablespoons sugar
1 teaspoon Asian sesame oil
Salt, to taste

8 ounces bay scallops
8 ounces medium-large shrimp, cooked and cut in half
1 cucumber, seeded and thinly sliced
8 Chinese dried black mushrooms, soaked in warm water for about 20 minutes, stems removed, caps julienned
1 red bell pepper, cut into 1 1/2-inch-long julienne
Salad greens
2 green onions, cut on the diagonal into 1/4-inch slices
1 tablespoon sesame seeds, lightly toasted (optional)

Heat a nonstick stir-fry pan or skillet over medium heat. Add the canola oil. Heat. Add the dried red chilies and stir until they turn brownish. Add the five-spice powder. Stir for just a few seconds to prevent the five-spice powder from burning. Add the chicken stock, soy sauce, red wine vinegar, and sugar. Stir until the sugar dissolves. Remove from the heat. Stir in the sesame oil. Season with salt. Set aside to cool. Remove and discard the dried chilies. Pour into a jar, cover, and refrigerate.

Rinse and drain the scallops. Place them on a steamer rack over boiling water. Cover and steam the scallops until they are just opaque, 4 to 5 minutes. Remove the steamer rack from the heat. Let the scallops cool. Cover and refrigerate.

When ready to serve, combine the shrimp, scallops, cucumber, mushrooms, and bell pepper in a large bowl. Shake the dressing and pour over the salad, tossing the salad ingredients to coat them with the dressing. Place the salad greens on a serving platter or individual plates and top with the salad. Sprinkle the salad with green onions and sesame seeds, if using.

*Yield: 4 servings*

| | | | |
|---|---|---|---|
| Calories | 261 | Cholesterol | 135 mg |
| Fat | 10 g | Sodium | 425 mg |
| Saturated Fat | 0 g | Carbohydrate | 19 g |
| Mono | 5 g | Protein | 25 g |
| Poly | 3 g | | |

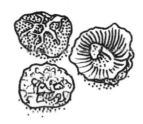

# TOMATOES STUFFED WITH SPICY CHICKEN SALAD

FOR AN attractive cocktail version, stuff halved cherry tomatoes.

The chicken may be prepared one day ahead and refrigerated, covered. Stuff the tomatoes no more than one hour before serving.

    4 medium, firm, ripe tomatoes
    1/4 teaspoon salt
    1 clove garlic, crushed
    1/2 pound boneless and skinless chicken breasts and thighs, ground
    1/4 cup fat-free low-sodium Chicken Stock (page 60) or water
    1 tablespoon minced shallot
    1/4 to 1 teaspoon red pepper powder
    2 teaspoons fish sauce
    1 green onion, coarsely chopped
    1 stalk fresh lemon grass, bottom 6 inches only, minced
    1 tablespoon chopped mint leaves
    1 tablespoon long-grain rice, toasted and ground
    2 tablespoons fresh lime juice
    Whole mint leaves, for garnish
    Lettuce leaves

Cut a thin slice off the stem end of each tomato. Scoop out the pulp and discard. Season the tomato shells lightly with salt and rub the inside of each tomato with the garlic clove. Invert on a rack to drain for about 15 minutes. Dry the inside of the tomatoes with a paper towel.

Heat a nonstick skillet over medium heat. Add the chicken and stock and cook, stirring, until the chicken is no longer pink. Add the shallot, red pepper powder, and fish sauce and cook for about 30 seconds. Remove from the heat. Add the green onion, lemon grass, mint leaves, ground rice, and lime juice. Toss to combine.

Fill the tomatoes with the mixture. Garnish with the mint leaves. Serve on a bed of lettuce leaves.

*Yield: 4 servings*

| | | | |
|---|---|---|---|
| Calories | 115 | Cholesterol | 34 mg |
| Fat | 2 g | Sodium | 300 mg |
| Saturated Fat | 0 g | Carbohydrate | 10 g |
| Mono | 1 g | Protein | 15 g |
| Poly | 0 g | | |

# VIETNAMESE SHRIMP SALAD

A SUBTLE blending of textures and light, aromatic flavors enhances this shrimp salad. Wrap it in a Boston lettuce leaf to make a package for an appetizer.

1/4 cup (loosely packed) fresh coriander (cilantro) leaves
8 ounces cooked medium shrimp, shelled and deveined
1/2 cup thinly sliced peeled and seeded cucumber
1/2 cup peeled and thinly sliced daikon
1/4 cup thinly sliced red onion
2 green onions, thinly sliced
1 tablespoon fish sauce
1 tablespoon rice vinegar
2 tablespoons fresh lime juice
2 teaspoons sugar
1 red chili, seeded and thinly sliced (optional)
2 tablespoons chopped unsalted dry-roasted peanuts (optional)

Chop all but 8 of the coriander leaves. Combine the chopped coriander, shrimp, cucumber, daikon, red onion, green onions, fish sauce, vinegar, lime juice, and sugar in a serving bowl. Toss lightly to combine. Cover and chill in the refrigerator. When ready to serve, garnish with fresh coriander leaves and chili and peanuts, if using.

*Yield: 4 servings*

| | | | |
|---|---|---|---|
| Calories | 82 | Cholesterol | 110 mg |
| Fat | 1 g | Sodium | 303 mg |
| Saturated Fat | 0 g | Carbohydrate | 6 g |
| Mono | 0 g | Protein | 13 g |
| Poly | 0 g | | |

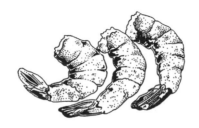

# BASMATI RICE AND VEGETABLE SALAD

RED TOMATOES and green cucumber lend a burst of color to this aromatic Indian basmati rice salad, which will be the highlight of your next buffet. Feel free to substitute diced red peppers and blanched shredded snow peas or any other colorful vegetables of your choice in this salad. Long-grain rice can be substituted but you will lose the distinctive nutty flavor of the basmati rice. If using long-grain rice, cook as directed on page 274. Serve this do-ahead salad in the summer with grilled poultry or fish or on a winter buffet with roasted chicken or steamed fish.

The dressing and rice may be prepared ahead. Toss immediately before serving.

1 cup basmati rice
2 tablespoons rice vinegar
3 tablespoons fresh lime juice
1 tablespoon extra virgin olive oil
1 clove garlic, crushed
1/8 to 1/4 teaspoon red pepper flakes, or to taste
Salt and freshly ground black pepper, to taste
2 cups seeded and diced (1/4-inch) ripe tomatoes
1 medium cucumber, seeded, and cut into 1/4-inch dice
3 tablespoons fresh coriander (cilantro), chopped
1/4 cup loosely packed chopped mint leaves
1 cup coarsely chopped water chestnuts (optional)
6 to 8 lettuce leaves
2 tablespoons chopped unsalted cashews, toasted (optional)
Sprigs of mint

Place the rice in a bowl. Cover with water. Rub the grains together between the palms of your hands until the water becomes cloudy. Pour the rice into a strainer to drain. Repeat the washing procedure 3 to 5 times or until the water is clear. Drain thoroughly. Put the rice in a bowl. Add water to cover the rice by at least 1 inch. Soak the rice for at least 20 minutes. Drain. (If using long-grain rice omit this procedure.)

Bring 2 cups water to a boil in a saucepan. Add the rice and bring to a boil. Cover the pan with a tight-fitting lid. Reduce the heat and simmer until all the water is absorbed, 15 to 18 minutes. Do not lift the lid. After 15 minutes, lift the lid just long enough to check to see that all the water is absorbed. When done, remove from the heat. Let the rice rest, covered, for at least 5 minutes. With chopsticks or a fork, fluff the rice. Let the rice cool before combining with the other ingredients.

Combine the vinegar, lime juice, oil, garlic, red pepper flakes, salt, and pepper in a large bowl. Whisk to blend. Add the tomatoes, cucumber, coriander, mint, and water chestnuts, if using. Toss to blend. Add the rice and toss to blend. Serve on lettuce leaves, garnished with cashews, if desired, and sprigs of mint.

*Yield: 6 servings*

| | | | |
|---|---|---|---|
| Calories | 149 | Cholesterol | 0 mg |
| Fat | 3 g | Sodium | 30 mg |
| Saturated Fat | 0 g | Carbohydrate | 28 g |
| Mono | 2 g | Protein | 4 g |
| Poly | 0 g | | |

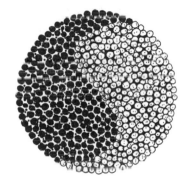

# JAPANESE SMOKED SALMON SALAD

MY FRIEND Akemi Ueki combines smoked salmon, cucumber, red onion, and lettuce in this chilled summer salad—a great overture for any dinner. She says that in Japan smoked salmon is almost always served with red onions.

1/4 red onion, thinly sliced
1/3 pound thinly sliced smoked salmon, cut into 1 1/2-inch pieces
2 stalks celery, thinly sliced on the diagonal
1/2 English or hothouse cucumber, cut in half lengthwise and thinly sliced on the
    diagonal
2 leaves romaine or other lettuce, torn into bite-size pieces

### Dressing
1 tablespoon canola oil
1 1/2 tablespoons rice vinegar
2 teaspoons low-sodium soy sauce
Salt and pepper, to taste

Rinse the red onion under cold water. Drain well. Combine the salmon, celery, cucumber, onion, and romaine in a serving bowl. Cover and chill.

Combine the dressing ingredients in a small bowl. Drizzle the dressing over the salad just before serving.

*Yield: 4 servings*

| | | | |
|---|---|---|---|
| Calories | 89 | Cholesterol | 9 mg |
| Fat | 5 g | Sodium | 402 mg |
| Saturated Fat | 1 g | Carbohydrate | 2 g |
| Mono | 3 g | Protein | 8 g |
| Poly | 1 g | | |

# THAI NOODLE AND VEGETABLE SALAD

DELICATELY FLAVORED rice noodles supply the perfect counterpoint for vegetables dressed with a zesty sauce with a hint of fire. Filipino-born Lilay Layaoen, specialist chef at the Princeville Resort on Kauai, who inspired this dish, serves it as a side dish with grilled fish or chicken. For a heartier salad, she suggests adding cooked shrimp or chicken.

8 ounces dried 1/4-inch rice noodles (rice vermicelli), soaked in warm water for
    20 minutes and drained
1 teaspoon Asian sesame oil
1/2 cup fresh bean sprouts
1/2 cucumber, cut lengthwise in half, seeded, and cut into 2-inch-long julienne
1 carrot, cut into 2-inch-long julienne
1/4 cup chopped green onion
1/4 cup chopped fresh coriander (cilantro) or mint
1 to 3 red chilies, seeded and minced, or 1/2 to 1 teaspoon red pepper flakes
1 clove garlic, minced
2 tablespoons rice vinegar
3 tablespoons fresh lime juice
2 tablespoons fish sauce, or to taste (optional)
2 tablespoons sugar
2 to 3 tablespoons chopped unsalted dry-roasted peanuts

Bring 4 quarts of water to a boil. Add the noodles and stir to separate. When the water returns to a boil, cook until just tender to the bite, 1 to 2 minutes. Drain the noodles. Toss with the oil.

    Toss the bean sprouts, cucumber, carrot, green onion, and half the fresh coriander into the noodles. Combine the chilies, garlic, vinegar, lime juice, fish sauce, and sugar in a bowl. Add to the vegetables and toss to combine. Garnish with the remaining coriander. Sprinkle peanuts over the top. Serve.

*Yield: 4 to 6 servings*

| Calories | 190 | Cholesterol | 0 mg |
|---|---|---|---|
| Fat | 2 g | Sodium | 9 mg |
| Saturated Fat | 0 g | Carbohydrate | 38 g |
| Mono | 1 g | Protein | 6 g |
| Poly | 0 g | | |

# SOBA NOODLE SALAD

JANICE MATSUMOTO, a longtime resident of Yokohama, combines flavorful soba (buckwheat noodles) with crunchy vegetables and a tart sesame-soy dressing in her Japanese salad.

### Dressing
¹/₄ cup *Dashi* (page 61)
2 tablespoons low-sodium soy sauce
¹/₄ cup rice vinegar
1 tablespoon sugar
1 teaspoon Asian sesame oil

7 ounces dried thin (200 grams) soba or ³/₄ pound fresh buckwheat noodles
7 ounces tofu (¹/₂ cake), drained and cut into ¹/₂ inch cubes (optional)
¹/₂ cup peeled and julienned daikon
1 cup radish sprouts
1 small onion, cut in half, thinly sliced, rinsed, and drained
2 tablespoons finely chopped green onion
1 tablespoon sesame seeds, toasted
Japanese seven-spice powder, to taste

Combine the dressing ingredients in a small bowl and set aside.

Bring 2 quarts of water to a boil in a large pot over high heat. Separate the noodles and drop them into the boiling water, stirring once or twice. When the water begins to boil over, add 1 cup of cold water. Repeat twice. Lower the heat and cook until the noodles are tender, about 3 to 4 minutes. Drain in a colander. Rinse with cold water until completely chilled, rubbing vigorously with hands to remove all surface starch. If using fresh soba, blanch the noodles in rapidly boiling water for 10 to 15 seconds. Drain thoroughly. Rinse as above.

Divide the noodles among 4 bowls. Arrange the tofu, if desired, daikon, sprouts, and onion on top of the noodles. Garnish with the green onion, sesame seeds, and a dash of seven-spice powder. Pour the dressing over the salad. Serve.

*Yield: 4 servings*

| | | | |
|---|---|---|---|
| Calories | 235 | Cholesterol | 0 mg |
| Fat | 3 g | Sodium | 663 mg |
| Saturated Fat | 0 g | Carbohydrate | 48 g |
| Mono | 1 g | Protein | 8 g |
| Poly | 1 g | | |

# SMALL DISHES

## SIDE DISHES

Carrot and Cabbage Slaw
Indian Spiced Mung Beans with Spinach (*Palak Moong Dal*)
Sweet and Spicy Lentils (*Gujarathi Dal*)
Hot-and-Sour Cucumbers
Indian Cucumber and Yogurt Raita
Japanese Cucumber Salad (*Sunomono*)
Japanese Pickled Daikon and Cucumber
Japanese Radish Salad
Spinach with Toasted Sesame Seed Dressing

## SALSAS, SAMBALS, AND CHUTNEYS

Padang-style Indonesian Salsa (*Acar Padang*)
Indonesian Red Chili Sambal (*Sambal Goreng*)
Thai Red Chili Salsa (*Nam Prik*)
Summer Cucumber and Daikon Kimchi
Spicy Thai Eggplant Salsa
Pineapple Salsa
Mango Salsa
Hawaiian Tropical Salsa
Papaya and Maui Onion Salsa
Mint-Coriander Chutney
Banana Relish

## DRESSINGS AND SAUCES

Orange-Ginger Dressing
Spicy Peanut Sauce
Coriander-Mint Dipping Sauce
Soy-Sesame-Orange Dipping Sauce
Soy-Vinegar-Sesame Dipping Sauce
Vietnamese Nuoc Cham Sauce
Japanese Ponzu Sauce

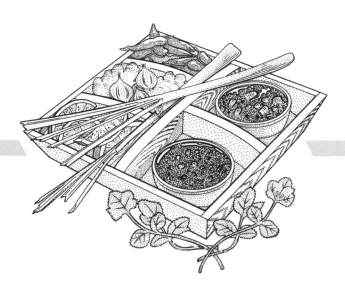

# SMALL DISHES

Essential small dishes add panache to Pacific Rim dining. I have become addicted to the intense, bold flavors that explode in your mouth from such fruit and/or vegetable accompaniments as Padang-style Indonesian Salsa, Spicy Thai Eggplant Salsa, Hawaiian Tropical Salsa, and Indonesian Red Chili Sambal. More subtle are Carrot and Cabbage Slaw, Hot-and-Sour Cucumbers, and Japanese Radish Salad.

Throughout the book I have suggested salsas or accompaniments to serve with individual dishes, but there are no rules. Let your imagination be your guide. A low-calorie, low-fat meal will never seem dull when served with one of these vivid, aromatic, and easily prepared salsas.

# CARROT AND CABBAGE SLAW

GINGER, GARLIC, and chilies lend this colorful slaw an Hawaiian emphasis. For a really quick slaw, purchase packaged sliced cabbage and grated carrots at the supermarket, add the remaining salad ingredients, and serve with the dressing.

4 carrots, julienned
4 cups thinly sliced Chinese or napa cabbage
1/2 cup red onion, minced
20 snow peas, strings removed and julienned (optional)

### Dressing
1 tablespoon peeled and minced fresh ginger
2 cloves garlic, minced
2 to 4 red chilies, seeded and finely chopped
2 tablespoons fresh lime juice
1 tablespoon rice vinegar
1/2 teaspoon sugar
1 tablespoon extra virgin olive oil
Salt and freshly ground black pepper, to taste

Combine the carrots, cabbage, onion, and snow peas, if using, in a large bowl and toss. In a small bowl, combine the ginger, garlic, chilies, lime juice, vinegar, sugar, oil, salt, and pepper. Pour over the slaw vegetables and toss. Serve immediately.

*Yield: 8 to 10 servings*

| Calories | 35 | Cholesterol | 0 mg |
|---|---|---|---|
| Fat | 1 g | Sodium | 15 mg |
| Saturated Fat | 0 g | Carbohydrate | 5 g |
| Mono | 1 g | Protein | 1 g |
| Poly | 0 g | | |

# INDIAN SPICED MUNG BEANS
# WITH SPINACH

## PALAK MOONG DAL

FRESH SPINACH and dried beans are laced with a spicy tomato-based mixture in this nutritious dal inspired by Savithri Lakshman, Consul at the Consulate General of India in Chicago. She says variations of this dal are served throughout India. Savithri serves it with rice as a vegetarian meal or with roti, an Indian flatbread. It can also be served as a side dish with a meal.

Savithri makes her dal saucy since she serves it with rice. I prefer a dryer dal. Choose the consistency you like, taking into account the texture of the other dishes served. The dal may be made thicker by reducing the amount of water used for cooking the beans. Add more water and adjust the seasonings for a soup.

She soaks the mung beans before cooking to reduce the cooking time. If you wish, you may cook the beans for one hour instead of soaking. If split mung beans are unavailable, Indian *chana dal* or supermarket yellow split peas can be substituted. Cook the peas for about forty-five minutes, or until tender.

> 1 cup split dried mung beans (*moong dal*)
> 1/8 teaspoon turmeric
> 1/2 pound spinach, washed, drained, and coarsely chopped, or 1 package
>     (10 ounces) frozen leaf spinach, defrosted
> 1 teaspoon canola oil
> 1/2 teaspoon cumin seeds
> 1/2 teaspoon red pepper powder, or to taste
> 1/2 teaspoon peeled and minced ginger
> 1/2 cup finely chopped tomatoes
> Salt, to taste
> 2 teaspoons fresh lemon juice
> 1/4 teaspoon freshly ground Garam Masala (page 278) (optional)

Pick the beans over carefully to remove any that are hard and any foreign matter. Put the beans in a fine-mesh sieve and lower it into a bowl full of water. Rub the beans between your hands. Remove and discard the water. Repeat the process until the water is clear. Place the beans in a bowl. Cover with 1 1/2 inches of water. Let the beans soak for 1 hour. Drain.

Combine the beans, 2 cups of water, and the turmeric in a heavy 3-quart saucepan over high heat. Bring to a boil. Reduce the heat to low. Cover with a tight-fitting lid and cook, skimming off any foam, for 7 to 10 minutes, or until the beans are tender and plump. It should not be cooked so long that it begins to fall apart. Add the spinach, and cook for 3 to 4 minutes, or until the spinach is cooked and has blended well with the beans.

Heat the oil in a small nonstick pan over medium heat. Add the cumin seeds and stir until dark brown, 10 to 15 seconds. Add the red pepper powder, ginger, and tomatoes. Stir for 1 minute. Add the cooked tomato mixture to the spinach and beans mixture. Season with salt and lemon juice. The dal will thicken upon standing. For additional flavor, sprinkle Garam Masala over the dal just before serving, if desired. Serve as a side dish or with rice.

*Yield: 4 to 6 servings*

| Calories | 133 | Cholesterol | 0 mg |
|----------|-----|-------------|------|
| Fat | 1 g | Sodium | 37 mg |
| Saturated Fat | 0 g | Carbohydrate | 22 g |
| Mono | 0 g | Protein | 9 g |
| Poly | 1 g | | |

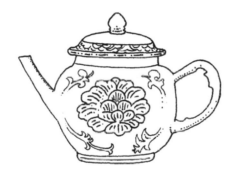

# SWEET AND SPICY LENTILS

## GUJARATHI DAL

WHILE VISITING Bombay, I had the good fortune to be interviewed by Anjali Joshi Reddy, a columnist and feature writer for the *Sunday Observer*, Bombay. Since then, she got married, and she now is my neighbor in Hinsdale, Illinois.

Her recipe for *Gujarathi Dal* from her home state of Gujarat is outstanding. A legume dish, or dal, is served daily in India, with rice or as part of a meal; it is a major source of protein. Anjali has perfectly combined the spices of India in this dish, blending spicy and sweet with a touch of lemon. She suggests adding additional water to the finished dish to make a soup. She also says you can add thinly sliced radishes for a more pungent aroma and taste.

Yellow lentils (*toor dal*, also known as *toovar dal* and *arhar dal*) are pale yellow to gold in color; they can be purchased in Indian grocery stores. Indian grocery stores also carry black mustard seeds and fresh curry leaves, which add a piquant aroma.

If toor dal is unavailable, substitute yellow split peas. Cook the peas for about forty-five minutes, or until tender.

    1 cup yellow lentils (toor dal)
    1/2 teaspoon turmeric
    1 teaspoon ground cumin
    1 teaspoon ground coriander
    1 green chili, seeded and finely chopped
    1 tablespoon canola oil
    1 teaspoon black mustard seeds
    7 to 8 fresh curry leaves (optional)
    1 small piece of ginger, peeled and minced
    1/2 teaspoon red pepper powder
    2 to 3 tablespoons brown sugar, or to taste
    1 teaspoon fresh lemon juice, or to taste
    Salt, to taste
    3 tablespoons finely chopped fresh coriander (cilantro) leaves, for garnish

Pick the lentils over carefully to remove any kernels that are too hard and for foreign matter. Put the lentils in a fine-mesh sieve and lower it into a bowl full of water. Rub between your hands. Remove and discard the water. Repeat until the water is clear.

Combine the lentils with 4 cups of water in a large, heavy-bottomed nonstick saucepan. Bring to a boil over high heat, skimming off any foam. Reduce the heat to medium-low and cook, covered, until soft and mushy, about 30 minutes. Stir occasionally to prevent burning.

The lentils are ready when they are tender and break easily when pressed between the thumb and index finger. Remove from the heat and beat the lentils with a wire whisk or an immersion blender until creamy and smooth. The mixture should be the consistency of a creamy soup. Add more water if needed.

Return the pan to the heat and add the turmeric, cumin, coriander, and chili. Simmer gently for 15 minutes, adding more water if the mixture starts to stick to the pan. Use a heat diffuser if necessary.

Heat the oil in a small pan over high heat. Add the mustard seeds. When they begin to pop, add the curry leaves, if using, ginger, and red pepper powder. Fry the spices for a minute and add them to the lentils. Add the brown sugar, lemon juice, and salt. Stir to blend. The consistency of the finished dish should be that of a creamy soup. If it is too thick, add more water.

When serving, garnish with the coriander. Serve as a side dish or Indian style, hot with plain rice.

*Yield: 4 to 6 servings*

| | | | |
|---|---|---|---|
| Calories | 170 | Cholesterol | 0 mg |
| Fat | 3 g | Sodium | 25 mg |
| Saturated Fat | 0 g | Carbohydrate | 30 g |
| Mono | 1 g | Protein | 1 g |
| Poly | 1 g | | |

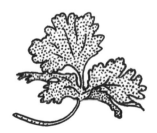

# HOT-AND-SOUR CUCUMBERS

CUCUMBER SALADS can be found almost everywhere in Southeast Asia. They are served with grilled and fried foods to tame the heat. These cucumbers are an excellent accompaniment to Thai Corn Cakes (page 18), Chicken Satay (page 104), and grilled seafood.

2 firm cucumbers, peeled, cut lengthwise in half, seeded, and thinly sliced
1/4 cup minced red onion
2 to 4 red chilies, seeded and thinly sliced
1/3 cup rice vinegar
2 teaspoons sugar
2 teaspoons minced fresh coriander (cilantro)
3 tablespoons coarsely chopped unsalted dry-roasted peanuts (optional)

Place the cucumbers in a serving bowl and toss with the onion, chilies, rice vinegar, and sugar. Garnish with coriander and chopped peanuts, if desired.

*Yield: 4 to 6 servings*

| | | | |
|---|---|---|---|
| Calories | 23 | Cholesterol | 0 mg |
| Fat | 0 g | Sodium | 3 mg |
| Saturated Fat | 0 g | Carbohydrate | 5 g |
| Mono | 0 g | Protein | 1 g |
| Poly | 0 g | | |

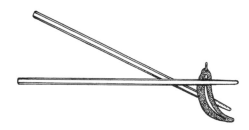

# INDIAN CUCUMBER AND YOGURT RAITA

THIS CLASSIC Indian yogurt salad is a cooling addition to a spicy meal. For a variation, serve it as a dip with vegetables. Traditionally made with whole-milk yogurt, raita works well with non-fat yogurt.

1 small cucumber, peeled, seeded, and diced
1/4 cup chopped red onion
1/2 teaspoon minced garlic (optional)
1 to 2 green chilies, seeded and minced
1 tablespoon chopped mint leaves
1 tablespoon fresh lemon juice
2 cups plain non-fat yogurt

Combine all the ingredients in a bowl and mix well. Serve.

*Yield: 4 to 6 servings*

| | | | |
|---|---|---|---|
| Calories | 53 | Cholesterol | 1 mg |
| Fat | 0 g | Sodium | 59 mg |
| Saturated Fat | 0 g | Carbohydrate | 8 g |
| Mono | 0 g | Protein | 4 g |
| Poly | 0 g | | |

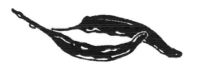

# JAPANESE CUCUMBER SALAD

## SUNOMONO

FROM TOD Kawachi, Executive Chef of Roy's Kahana Restaurant on Maui, comes this simple traditional salad, which has been served for more than a thousand years in Japan and which is still an important element of a Japanese meal. This is a palate refresher for any occasion. Chef Kawachi feels the sweet pink and the spicy red pickled gingers provide an interesting juxtaposition of flavors.

1 medium cucumber, peeled, seeded, and cut into paper-thin slices
Salt
2 tablespoons thinly julienned carrot
2 tablespoons thinly sliced pink pickled ginger
2 tablespoons sliced red pickled ginger
1/4 cup thinly sliced red or Maui onion
1 cup rice vinegar
2 tablespoons sugar
Watercress leaves, for garnish

Sprinkle the cucumbers lightly with salt. Allow to stand for 10 minutes. Squeeze with your hands to remove excess liquid. Rinse with cold water and gently squeeze dry.

Toss the cucumber, carrot, pink and red pickled gingers, onion, rice vinegar, and sugar in a bowl. Refrigerate for at least 1 hour. Serve chilled, garnished with watercress leaves.

*Yield: 4 to 6 servings*

| | | | |
|---|---|---|---|
| Calories | 40 | Cholesterol | 0 mg |
| Fat | 0 g | Sodium | 53 mg |
| Saturated Fat | 0 g | Carbohydrate | 10 g |
| Mono | 0 g | Protein | 1 g |
| Poly | 0 g | | |

# JAPANESE PICKLED DAIKON AND CUCUMBER

PICKLED VEGETABLES appear on many Japanese tables throughout the year. Particularly refreshing when served with hot-pot dishes such as *Yudofu*, *Yosenabe*, and *Shabu Shabu* (pages 127–133), the pickles go with almost any Asian meal.

Use only daikon or only cucumber if you like. The pickles will keep, tightly covered, in the refrigerator for about one month.

### Dressing
$^1/_2$ cup rice vinegar
$^1/_4$ cup sugar
Salt, to taste
Dash of Japanese seven-spice powder

1 to 2 small daikons, peeled, quartered, and thinly sliced, about 2 cups
$^1/_2$ cucumber, seeded and thinly sliced
2 teaspoons salt

Combine the vinegar, sugar, and salt in a small saucepan over low heat. Cook, stirring, until the sugar dissolves. Add the seven-spice powder. Let cool.

Sprinkle the daikon and cucumber slices with salt and let stand for 10 minutes. Squeeze with your hands to remove liquid. Discard the liquid. Rinse with cold water and gently squeeze dry.

Tightly pack the vegetables in a wide-mouthed jar and pour the dressing over them. Cover the jar and let stand at room temperature for at least 2 hours or in the refrigerator for at least 8 hours before serving. Keep refrigerated.

*Yield: 4 to 6 servings*

| | | | |
|---|---|---|---|
| Calories | 46 | Cholesterol | 0 mg |
| Fat | 0 g | Sodium | 52 mg |
| Saturated Fat | 0 g | Carbohydrate | 12 g |
| Mono | 0 g | Protein | 1 g |
| Poly | 0 g | | |

# JAPANESE RADISH SALAD

A SWEET-AND-SOUR dressing complements brilliant red radishes in Akemi Ueki's salad. For a variation, add half a cucumber, peeled, seeded, and diced. Serve with *Shabu Shabu* (page 127) or grilled fish or chicken.

1 large bunch red radishes, trimmed and thinly sliced
1 1/2 teaspoons rice vinegar
1 teaspoon sugar
1/2 teaspoon low-sodium soy sauce
2 teaspoons sesame seeds, toasted (optional)
Radish leaves, for garnish (optional)

Combine the radishes, vinegar, sugar, and soy sauce in a small serving bowl. Refrigerate for 1 hour. When ready to serve, sprinkle with sesame seeds and garnish with radish leaves, if desired.

*Yield: 4 servings*

| Calories | 12 | Cholesterol | 0 mg |
| Fat | 0 g | Sodium | 32 mg |
| Saturated Fat | 0 g | Carbohydrate | 2 g |
| Mono | 0 g | Protein | 0 g |
| Poly | 0 g | | |

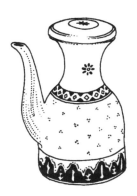

# SPINACH WITH TOASTED SESAME SEED DRESSING

GROUND TOASTED sesame seeds impart a nutty flavor to this salad, which is served in almost every Japanese home and restaurant. For best results, use the young, tender, fresh spinach leaves sold in bunches. Be sure not to overcook the spinach. It should be barely wilted.

2 tablespoons sesame seeds, toasted
1 tablespoon sugar
2 1/2 tablespoons low-sodium soy sauce
1 pound fresh spinach, stemmed and washed

In a blender or mini food processor, process the sesame seeds until flaky. Add the sugar and soy sauce and process just to combine.

Bring a large saucepan of water to a boil and blanch the spinach for 30 seconds, or until it barely wilts. Drain and refresh in cold water. Squeeze out the excess moisture and coarsely chop the leaves.

Toss the spinach with the sesame seed dressing. Serve chilled or at room temperature.

*Yield: 4 servings*

| | | | |
|---|---|---|---|
| Calories | 69 | Cholesterol | 0 mg |
| Fat | 3 g | Sodium | 420 mg |
| Saturated Fat | 0 g | Carbohydrate | 9 g |
| Mono | 1 g | Protein | 5 g |
| Poly | 1 g | | |

# SALSAS, SAMBALS, AND CHUTNEYS

# PADANG-STYLE INDONESIAN SALSA

## ACAR PADANG

THE PEOPLE of Padang, West Sumatra, like their food fiery hot, especially their condiments. I have toned down this salsa to suit American tastes. If you prefer to have your *acar* real Padang style, just add more chilies. Acar is best made a day ahead and served chilled or at room temperature. Serve it with grilled meat, fish, or chicken or as a palate refresher with Asian or Western foods.

The salsa will keep, tightly covered, in the refrigerator for three to four days.

1 tablespoon canola oil
6 cloves garlic, chopped
1 tablespoon peeled and minced fresh ginger
1 teaspoon ground cumin
1 teaspoon ground nutmeg
1 teaspoon turmeric
1 teaspoon ground coriander
$1/2$ cup rice vinegar
$1/4$ cup (firmly packed) light brown sugar
3 carrots, cut into $1^1/2$-inch-long julienne
1 cucumber, seeded and cut into $1^1/2$-inch-long julienne
1 red bell pepper, quartered, seeded, and cut into very thin slices
2 to 4 red chilies, seeded and chopped
Salt, to taste
2 tablespoons fresh lime juice
3 tablespoons chopped fresh coriander (cilantro) leaves

Heat the oil in a large nonstick skillet over medium heat. Add the garlic and ginger. Cook, stirring frequently to prevent burning, until light brown, about 2 minutes. Add the cumin, nutmeg, turmeric, and coriander. Cook for about 30 seconds, stirring to prevent burning. Add the vinegar and brown sugar and stir for about 2 minutes. Add the carrots, cucumber, bell pepper, and chilies and toss thoroughly to combine. Remove from the heat. Season with salt. Let the mixture cool.

Stir in the lime juice and chopped coriander leaves, reserving some for garnish. Place the mixture in a glass container. Refrigerate, tightly covered, overnight, to allow flavors to blend. Sprinkle reserved chopped coriander on top. Serve chilled or at room temperature.

*Yield: about 2 cups*

| Calories | 39 | Cholesterol | 0 mg |
|---|---|---|---|
| Fat | 1 g | Sodium | 7 mg |
| Saturated Fat | 0 g | Carbohydrate | 8 g |
| Mono | 0 g | Protein | 1 g |
| Poly | 0 g | | |

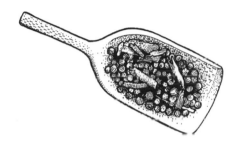

# INDONESIAN RED CHILI SAMBAL

## SAMBAL GORENG

SAMBALS CONTAIN almost no cholesterol or fat and are served as a side dish to add intensity to almost any dish. Their spicy heat will give the pizzazz to add adventure to your meal. This basic sambal was inspired by Joelina Soejono, wife of the Consul General of Indonesia in Chicago. If the sambal is too hot for your taste, Joelina suggests adding more ripe tomato.

The sambal can be stored, tightly covered, in the refrigerator for about one week.

15 to 18 long red chilies, seeded and coarsely chopped (about 4 ounces)
2 tablespoons chopped ripe tomato, or to taste
1 shallot, minced
1 teaspoon canola oil
Salt, to taste

In a mortar, mini food processor, or blender, pound or process the chilies, tomato, shallot, and 2 teaspoons water to a paste.

Heat the oil in a small nonstick skillet over medium heat. Add the paste mixture and cook, stirring, for about 2 minutes, adding water a tablespoon at a time if the paste starts to burn or stick to the pan. Season with salt.

*Yield: about 1 cup*

| | | | |
|---|---|---|---|
| Calories | 6 | Cholesterol | 0 mg |
| Fat | 0 g | Sodium | 1 mg |
| Saturated Fat | 0 g | Carbohydrate | 1 g |
| Mono | 0 g | Protein | 0 g |
| Poly | 0 g | | |

# THAI RED CHILI SALSA

## NAM PRIK

*NAM PRIK* is on the table during every Thai meal, and each family has its own rendition. It is so important to the Thais that the cooking ability of a cook is often judged on his or her Nam Prik. The sauce should be hot, sweet, and tangy. Adjust the sugar, fish sauce, and lime juice to your taste. Nam Prik is best made a day ahead. It will keep, tightly covered, in the refrigerator for several weeks.

    4 to 6 red chilies, seeded and chopped
    2 tablespoons dried shrimp, chopped
    6 cloves garlic, chopped
    1 tablespoon brown sugar, or to taste
    3 tablespoons fish sauce, or to taste
    3 tablespoons fresh lime juice, or to taste

In a mortar or mini processor, pound or process the chilies, dried shrimp, and garlic to a paste. Add the brown sugar, fish sauce, and lime juice. Adjust the seasonings. Refrigerate, tightly covered, for at least 1 day.

*Yield: 3/4 cup*

| | | | |
|---|---|---|---|
| Calories | 15 | Cholesterol | 1 mg |
| Fat | 0 g | Sodium | 175 mg |
| Saturated Fat | 0 g | Carbohydrate | 3 g |
| Mono | 0 g | Protein | 1 g |
| Poly | 0 g | | |

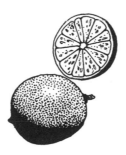

# SUMMER CUCUMBER AND DAIKON KIMCHI

KIMCHI IS a staple of the Korean diet and is consumed at every meal. It is considered Korea's national vegetable dish. The preparation of kimchi takes place in late fall. From grandmothers to small children, family members unite for the monumental task of making kimchi. Salt is used to prepare napa cabbage or other vegetables for fermentation. Then, daikons, cucumbers, or other vegetables, also pickled in brine, are added. Weeks of slow fermentation bring the blend to perfection. In the countryside, it is stored in large earthenware jars that are buried in the ground with only the covered opening of the jar above the ground, protecting it from the cold winter's snow.

In summer, kimchi prepared from red chili peppers and vegetables is made daily. Here is an easy summer kimchi made with cucumbers instead of the usual cabbage. Chung Hea Han, author of *Korean Cooking*, demonstrated this dish for me in her Seoul cooking school. You can serve the kimchi as a salad or as a condiment with both Asian and Western meals.

2 medium cucumbers, cut crosswise into 2-inch-long pieces
1 1/2 tablespoons salt
3/4 to 1 teaspoon red pepper powder
3 red chilies, seeded and minced
1 small daikon, cut into 1-inch-long julienne (about 2 cups)
2 green onions, cut into 1-inch-long julienne
1 small carrot, cut into 1-inch-long julienne
1 tablespoon peeled and minced fresh ginger
4 cloves garlic, minced
1 tablespoon sugar

Stand each cucumber piece on end. Cut a cross down each cucumber almost to the end. (Do not cut the ends. The cucumber section must remain whole.)

Dissolve the salt in enough water to cover the cucumbers. Soak the cucumbers in the salted water for 2 hours. This will allow them to become pliable for stuffing. Remove the cucumbers from the water. Squeeze out as much water as possible.

Meanwhile, combine the red pepper powder, chilies, daikon, green onions, carrot, ginger, garlic, and sugar in a large bowl. Set aside.

Stuff the cucumber slits with the daikon mixture as tightly as possible. Stand the cucumbers on end in a glass jar with a lid, stuffing any remaining daikon mixture between the cucumbers. Cover and place in a cool (about 60 degrees) dark place for 24 hours, turning occasionally. Refrigerate. The kimchi can be stored in the refrigerator for up to 4 days. To serve, cut into small pieces. Pour a little of the juice over the kimchi.

*Yield: about 5 cups*

| | | | |
|---|---|---|---|
| Calories | 6 | Cholesterol | 0 mg |
| Fat | 0 g | Sodium | 26 mg |
| Saturated Fat | 0 g | Carbohydrate | 1 g |
| Mono | 0 g | Protein | 1 g |
| Poly | 0 g | | |

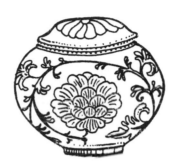

# SPICY THAI EGGPLANT SALSA

WELL SPICED and refreshing, this salsa is a stand-out addition to any Asian meal, and it goes with Western-style fish or chicken from the grill as well. Head chef Boon Choo Pho-lawatana of the Spice Market Restaurant in the Regent of Bangkok suggests using the small, slender Japanese eggplants for best results.

> Olive oil spray
> 1 Japanese eggplant, cut into $1/4$-inch cubes (about 1 pound)
> $1/4$ cup rice vinegar
> 2 teaspoons Asian sesame oil
> 1 tablespoon peeled and minced fresh ginger
> 1 teaspoon minced garlic
> 1 tablespoon fish sauce
> 1 tablespoon sugar
> 2 small red bell peppers, seeded and diced
> 1 medium red onion, diced
> 1 to 2 jalapeños, seeded and minced
> $1/3$ cup mint or fresh coriander (cilantro) leaves, chopped
> Salt and freshly ground black pepper, to taste

Preheat the oven to 450 degrees. Lightly oil or mist a baking sheet.

Spread the eggplant evenly on the baking sheet. Roast until the eggplant is soft, about 10 to 15 minutes. Remove from the oven. Let cool.

Combine the vinegar, sesame oil, ginger, garlic, fish sauce, and sugar in a large bowl. Stir until the sugar is dissolved. Add the roasted eggplant, bell peppers, onion, jalapeños, and mint, and toss to combine. Season with salt and pepper. Let stand at room temperature for 30 minutes before serving.

*Yield: 4 to 6 servings*

| | | | |
|---|---|---|---|
| Calories | 86 | Cholesterol | 0 mg |
| Fat | 2 g | Sodium | 130 mg |
| Saturated Fat | 0 g | Carbohydrate | 17 g |
| Mono | 1 g | Protein | 3 g |
| Poly | 1 g | | |

# PINEAPPLE SALSA

EXECUTIVE CHEF Daniel Delbrel of the Princeville Hotel on Kauai inspired this and the next colorful salsa, both of which can be served with grilled seafood or poultry. For an extra punch, he adds a seeded and chopped fresh red chili.

The salsa will keep, covered, in the refrigerator for two days.

1 cup diced ($1/4$ inch) ripe pineapple
$1/2$ cup diced ($1/4$ inch) green bell pepper
$1/2$ cup diced ($1/4$ inch) red bell pepper
$1/4$ cup coarsely chopped red onion
2 tablespoons chopped coriander (cilantro) leaves
2 tablespoons chopped green onions, green portion only
2 teaspoons fresh lemon juice
$1/2$ teaspoon fish sauce
2 teaspoons extra virgin olive oil (optional)
Salt and white pepper, to taste

Combine all the ingredients in a bowl. Let stand for 30 minutes before serving.

*Yield: about 2 1/2 cups*

| Calories | 8 | Cholesterol | 0 mg |
|---|---|---|---|
| Fat | 0 g | Sodium | 6 mg |
| Saturated Fat | 0 g | Carbohydrate | 2 g |
| Mono | 0 g | Protein | 0 g |
| Poly | 0 g | | |

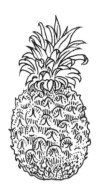

# MANGO SALSA

EXECUTIVE CHEF Daniel Delbrel says you may substitute peaches or pineapple for the mangoes.

The salsa will keep, covered, in the refrigerator for two days.

1 ripe mango (about 1 pound)
1 small red bell pepper, seeded and cut into julienne
1 tablespoon peeled and minced fresh ginger
1 red chili, seeded and finely chopped (optional)
1/2 cup thinly sliced red onion
2 tablespoons chopped fresh coriander (cilantro) leaves
5 tablespoons fresh lime juice
1/4 cup fresh orange or pineapple juice
Salt and white pepper, to taste

Peel the mango and cut it into 1/4-inch dice. Combine all of the ingredients in a bowl. Let stand at room temperature for 30 minutes before serving.

*Yield: about 3 cups*

| | | | |
|---|---|---|---|
| Calories | 17 | Cholesterol | 0 mg |
| Fat | 0 g | Sodium | 1 mg |
| Saturated Fat | 0 g | Carbohydrate | 4 g |
| Mono | 0 g | Protein | 0 g |
| Poly | 0 g | | |

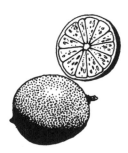

# HAWAIIAN TROPICAL SALSA

THIS SALSA is served everywhere in the Hawaiian islands. Brimming with bright fruit flavors and a touch of heat, it can be served with grilled seafood and chicken. If mangoes are unavailable, use ripe peaches or a combination of the ripest fruits of the season. Fresh mint may be substituted for the fresh coriander.

    1 large ripe mango (about 1 pound), peeled and cut into $1/4$-inch dice
    1 cup peeled and cored ripe pineapple wedges ($1/4$ inch thick)
    1 red bell pepper, quartered, seeded, and cut into $1/4$-inch slices
    1 small red onion, finely chopped
    1 green chili, seeded and finely chopped
    2 tablespoons finely chopped fresh coriander (cilantro) leaves
    1 teaspoon fresh lime juice
    Salt and freshly ground black pepper, to taste

Combine all of the ingredients in a medium bowl. Let stand at room temperature for 30 minutes before serving.

*Yield: about 3 cups*

| | | | |
|---|---|---|---|
| Calories | 15 | Cholesterol | 0 mg |
| Fat | 0 g | Sodium | 3 mg |
| Saturated Fat | 0 g | Carbohydrate | 4 g |
| Mono | 0 g | Protein | 0 g |
| Poly | 0 g | | |

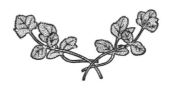

# PAPAYA AND MAUI ONION SALSA

THIS SPARKLING blend of papaya, citrus, and Maui onion is an adaptation of a salsa served by Executive Chef George Mavrothalassitis of La Mer Restaurant in the Halekulani Hotel in Honolulu. He serves it with grilled fish and chicken. I think it goes with almost anything. You can substitute many fruits, such as ripe mango and pineapple.

1 firm ripe papaya
$^1/_2$ cup chopped sweet onion, such as Maui, Walla Walla, or Vidalia
1 tablespoon peeled and minced fresh ginger
2 tablespoons chopped fresh coriander (cilantro) leaves
3 tablespoons fresh lime juice
1 tablespoon red wine vinegar
$^1/_8$ teaspoon red pepper powder (optional)

Peel the papaya and cut in half. Remove the seeds and cut into $^1/_4$-inch dice. Combine the papaya, onion, ginger, coriander, lime juice, vinegar, and red pepper powder, if using, in a bowl. Let stand at room temperature for 30 minutes before serving.

*Yield: about 1 cup*

| | | | |
|---|---|---|---|
| Calories | 50 | Cholesterol | 0 mg |
| Fat | 0 g | Sodium | 6 mg |
| Saturated Fat | 0 g | Carbohydrate | 12 g |
| Mono | 0 g | Protein | 1 g |
| Poly | 0 g | | |

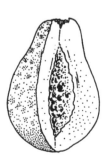

# MINT-CORIANDER CHUTNEY

IN INDIA, this chutney is made fresh daily. It is served with almost every meal. Try it with grilled seafood and poultry. When thinned with plain non-fat yogurt, it is an excellent dip for vegetables.

   1/2 cup (tightly packed) fresh mint leaves, coarsely chopped
   1/2 cup (tightly packed) fresh coriander (cilantro) leaves, coarsely chopped
   2 teaspoons peeled and chopped fresh ginger
   1/2 to 1 green chili, seeded and minced
   1 tablespoon fresh lemon juice
   Salt and freshly ground black pepper, to taste

Combine all the ingredients in a mini processor or blender. Process to a coarse paste. Place in a glass or other non-metallic container. Cover and refrigerate until ready to serve.

*Yield: about 1 cup*

| | | | |
|---|---|---|---|
| Calories | 3 | Cholesterol | 0 mg |
| Fat | 0 g | Sodium | 1 mg |
| Saturated Fat | 0 g | Carbohydrate | 1 g |
| Mono | 0 g | Protein | 0 g |
| Poly | 0 g | | |

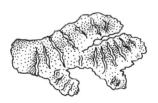

# BANANA RELISH

GRILLED FISH, chicken, and duck will be made more memorable when served with this spicy banana relish from Amy Ferguson Ota, Executive Chef of the Ritz-Carlton on Mauna Lani. She says it should have a balance of sweet and sour, curry, spice, and banana. She also likes the taste of Thai yellow curry paste, available in Asian grocery stores, as a change from the Madras curry powder.

1 teaspoon olive oil
1 large clove garlic, coarsely chopped
1 large shallot, coarsely chopped
1 teaspoon Madras curry powder
2 ripe bananas, peeled and coarsely chopped
$1/3$ cup fat-free low-sodium Chicken Stock (page 60)
1 teaspoon rice vinegar
$1/4$ teaspoon fresh lime juice
Salt and freshly ground black pepper, to taste
$1^1/2$ teaspoons honey (optional)

Heat the oil a nonstick skillet over medium heat. Add the garlic, shallot, and curry powder. Cook, stirring, for about 1 minute. Add the bananas and sauté for 1 minute more. Add the broth and cook over medium-high heat, stirring frequently, for about 3 to 5 minutes, or until the bananas are soft but not mushy and have formed a slightly thick, coarse puree. (The mixture will thicken more as it cools.) Season with vinegar, lime juice, salt, and pepper. If desired, add honey to balance flavors. Put in a bowl. Serve warm or at room temperature.

*Yield: $3/4$ cup*

| | | | |
|---|---|---|---|
| Calories | 71 | Cholesterol | 0 mg |
| Fat | 1 g | Sodium | 57 mg |
| Saturated Fat | 0 g | Carbohydrate | 15 g |
| Mono | 1 g | Protein | 2 g |
| Poly | 0 g | | |

# DRESSINGS AND SAUCES

# ORANGE-GINGER DRESSING

CRUSHED PAPAYA seeds add texture and a peppery taste to the orange and ginger in this unique Hawaiian dressing. Use the dressing on salad greens and fruit salads.

The dressing may be stored, tightly covered, in the refrigerator for up to 1 week.

$^3/_4$ teaspoon coarsely chopped shallot
1 teaspoon rinsed papaya seeds, crushed
1 teaspoon peeled and coarsely chopped fresh ginger
1 teaspoon Dijon mustard
$^2/_3$ cup fresh orange juice
2 tablespoons extra virgin olive oil
$^3/_4$ teaspoon Asian sesame oil
Salt, to taste

In a mini processor or blender, process the shallots, papaya seeds, ginger, mustard, and 2 tablespoons of the orange juice. Add the remaining orange juice, $^1/_4$ cup water, and olive and sesame oils and blend until emulsified. Season with salt. Refrigerate for at least 1 hour before serving. Shake well before using.

*Yield: about $^2/_3$ cup*

| | | | |
|---|---|---|---|
| Calories | 33 | Cholesterol | 0 mg |
| Fat | 3 g | Sodium | 6 mg |
| Saturated Fat | 0 g | Carbohydrate | 2 g |
| Mono | 2 g | Protein | 0 g |
| Poly | 0 g | | |

# SPICY PEANUT SAUCE

A GINGERY peanut sauce is often served in Indonesia with grilled meat, especially satays (page 104). When thinned with evaporated skim milk, it can be used as a dipping sauce for vegetables or as a salad dressing.

You can make the sauce several days ahead. It will thicken and mellow upon standing in the refrigerator. Stir in some evaporated skim milk or water when you reheat it. If you want to liven up the flavor, stir in more lime juice and red pepper.

2 teaspoons canola oil
1½ tablespoons peeled and minced ginger
1 tablespoon minced garlic
1 teaspoon red pepper flakes
1 tablespoon light soy sauce
2 tablespoons fresh lime juice
1 cup low-fat crunchy peanut butter
1 teaspoon brown sugar
⅛ teaspoon coconut flavoring
½ to ¾ cup evaporated skim milk

Heat the oil in a small nonstick pan. Add the ginger, garlic, and red pepper flakes. Stir for 30 seconds. Remove from the heat. Whisk in the soy sauce, lime juice, peanut butter, and brown sugar. Blend until well mixed. Cool. Add the coconut flavoring and as much evaporated skim milk as needed to thin to desired consistency. The sauce will thicken upon standing. Refrigerate until ready to serve.

*Yield: about 1⅓ cups*

| | | | |
|---|---|---|---|
| Calories | 164 | Cholesterol | 0 mg |
| Fat | 10 g | Sodium | 200 mg |
| Saturated Fat | 2 g | Carbohydrate | 10 g |
| Mono | 5 g | Protein | 8 g |
| Poly | 3 g | | |

# CORIANDER-MINT DIPPING SAUCE

SERVE THIS tangy all-purpose sauce with Thai Corn Cakes (page 18) or Chinese Pearl Balls, *Shao Mai*, Potstickers (pages 22–27), and other dumplings.

2 tablespoons fish sauce
6 tablespoons fresh lime juice
2 tablespoons rice vinegar
4 teaspoons sugar, or to taste
1 tablespoon peeled and minced ginger
4 teaspoons chopped fresh coriander (cilantro)
4 teaspoons chopped fresh mint
1 red chili, seeded and minced, or $1/4$ teaspoon red pepper flakes (optional)

In a bowl, combine the fish sauce, lime juice, vinegar, sugar, ginger, coriander, mint, and chili, if using. Stir until the sugar dissolves.

*Yield: about $2/3$ cup*

| | | | |
|---|---|---|---|
| Calories | 28 | Cholesterol | 0 mg |
| Fat | 0 g | Sodium | 277 mg |
| Saturated Fat | 0 g | Carbohydrate | 7 g |
| Mono | 0 g | Protein | 1 g |
| Poly | 0 g | | |

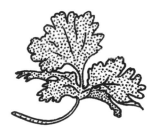

# SOY-SESAME-ORANGE DIPPING SAUCE

THIS VERSATILE dipping sauce is an excellent accompaniment to many dishes in this book, including *Shao Mai* and Potstickers (pages 22–27).

1 tablespoon low-sodium soy sauce
2 teaspoons red wine vinegar
$^1/_3$ cup fat-free low-sodium Chicken Stock (page 60)
3 tablespoons fresh orange juice
2 teaspoons peeled and minced fresh ginger
1 tablespoon minced mint or fresh coriander (cilantro) leaves
2 to 3 teaspoons hot sesame oil

Combine all the ingredients in a bowl. Serve.

*Yield: about $^3/_4$ cup*

| | | | |
|---|---|---|---|
| Calories | 11 | Cholesterol | 0 mg |
| Fat | 1 g | Sodium | 63 mg |
| Saturated Fat | 0 g | Carbohydrate | 1 g |
| Mono | 0 g | Protein | 0 g |
| Poly | 0 g | | |

# SOY-VINEGAR-SESAME DIPPING SAUCE

THIS SPIRITED Chinese sauce is another versatile dipping sauce perfect for Potstickers and *Shao Mai* (pages 22–25).

    ¹/₂ cup low-sodium soy sauce
    ¹/₂ cup water
    6 tablespoons rice vinegar
    2 to 3 teaspoons hot sesame oil

Combine all the ingredients in a bowl. Serve.

*Yield: about 1¹/₄ cups*

| | | | |
|---|---|---|---|
| Calories | 11 | Cholesterol | 0 mg |
| Fat | 0 g | Sodium | 392 mg |
| Saturated Fat | 0 g | Carbohydrate | 1 g |
| Mono | 0 g | Protein | 1 g |
| Poly | 0 g | | |

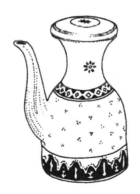

# VIETNAMESE NUOC CHAM SAUCE

THIS SAUCE is as common on Vietnamese tables as salt on American tables. It is a traditional accompaniment to spring rolls and Vietnamese Grilled Beef in Lettuce Packages (page 116). If the sauce is too strong for your taste, dilute it with a little water.

Nuoc Cham can be refrigerated, in a covered glass container, for up to one week.

2 tablespoons rice vinegar
3 tablespoons fresh lime juice
1/4 cup fish sauce
2 tablespoons sugar
1 clove garlic, minced
1 to 2 red chilies, seeded and minced
1 tablespoon fine carrot shreds, cut into 1 1/2-inch lengths

Combine the vinegar, lime juice, fish sauce, 1/4 cup water, and sugar in a bowl. Stir until the sugar dissolves. Add the garlic and chilies. Stir to combine. Sprinkle the carrot shreds on top. Cover and let stand at room temperature for 1 hour to blend flavors.

*Yield: 1 cup*

| | | | |
|---|---|---|---|
| Calories | 13 | Cholesterol | 0 mg |
| Fat | 0 g | Sodium | 173 mg |
| Saturated Fat | 0 g | Carbohydrate | 3 g |
| Mono | 0 g | Protein | 1 g |
| Poly | 0 g | | |

# JAPANESE PONZU SAUCE

CYRUS TAMISHIRO of Tamishiro's Market in Honolulu gave me his version of this flavorful dipping sauce. Often the sauce is made only with lemon juice, but Chef Tamishiro feels the addition of orange juice softens the harsh flavor of lemon when it is served with hot foods. Serve with such one-pot dishes as *Shabu Shabu*, *Yosenabe*, and *Yudofu* (pages 130–133).

3 tablespoons fresh lemon juice
1 tablespoon fresh orange juice
1/4 cup low-sodium soy sauce
2 tablespoons mirin

Combine all the ingredients. Serve.

*Yield: about 3/4 cup*

| | | | |
|---|---|---|---|
| Calories | 8 | Cholesterol | 0 mg |
| Fat | 0 g | Sodium | 212 mg |
| Saturated Fat | 0 g | Carbohydrate | 1 g |
| Mono | 0 g | Protein | 1 g |
| Poly | 0 g | | |

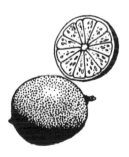

# DESSERTS AND BEVERAGES

## DESSERTS

Summer Fruits in Sweet Wine

Spiced Fruit Medley

Tropical Grilled Fruits with Lime Yogurt Sauce

Chinese Poached Pears

Orange-glazed Pears

*Haupia* with Tropical Fruits

Almond Float with Raspberry Sauce

Japanese Lemon Snow (*Awayukikan*)

Spiced Banana in a Banana Leaf

## BEVERAGES

Mango Refresher

Lemon Grass Mint Tea

Ginger Tea

Minted Green Tea

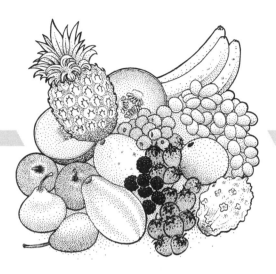

# DESSERTS AND BEVERAGES

WHILE SEASONED fresh fruit is often served at the beginning and during a meal in Asia, it is also common as an ending. That is not to say there aren't prepared desserts from countries around the Pacific. In this chapter are some of those I've found and enjoyed.

Easily prepared seasonal specialties include Summer Fruits in Sweet Wine, Chinese Poached Pears, Orange-glazed Pears, and Hawaiian almond-flavored *Haupia* with Tropical Fruits. All Southeast Asians enjoy Spiced Banana in a Banana Leaf grilled over an open fire. And, to me, Japanese Lemon Snow is the perfect finale to any dish in this collection.

# DESSERTS

# SUMMER FRUITS IN SWEET WINE

AMBROSIAL FRESH fruits luxuriating in a sea of cool sweet wine is a refreshing ending to a summer meal. You may substitute any fresh, colorful fruits in season. Executive Chef Daniel Delbrel of the Princeville Hotel on Kauai, who inspired this dish, also serves this often as a refreshing starter.

$1/2$ small ripe cantaloupe, seeded
1 firm ripe papaya, peeled, seeded, and sliced
1 ripe mango, peeled and sliced
24 raspberries
24 strawberries
1 cup sweet dessert wine, such as late harvest Riesling

Scoop out cantaloupe balls, using a 1-inch melon baller. Combine the cantaloupe, papaya, mango, raspberries, and strawberries in a bowl. Add the wine and toss gently. Cover and refrigerate overnight. To serve, arrange the fruit in wine goblets. Spoon the liquid over the fruit.

*Yield: 4 to 6 servings*

| | | | |
|---|---|---|---|
| Calories | 186 | Cholesterol | 0 mg |
| Fat | 1 g | Sodium | 31 mg |
| Saturated Fat | 0 g | Carbohydrate | 35 g |
| Mono | 0 g | Protein | 2 g |
| Poly | 0 g | | |

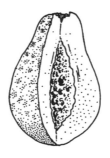

# SPICED FRUIT MEDLEY

SOUTHEAST ASIANS and Indians have a talent for tasty combinations of fresh fruits with unexpected spiced nuances. You may serve this as a dessert or as a palate cleanser during the meal.

1 large ripe papaya, peeled, seeded, and cut into $1/4$-inch pieces
2 ripe bananas, sliced
2 ripe pears, peeled, cored, and cut crosswise into $1/4$-inch pieces
$1/2$ ripe pineapple, peeled, cored, and cut into 1-inch pieces
2 small oranges, peeled, pith removed, and sectioned
$1/2$ cup unsweetened coconut flakes (optional)
$1/2$ cup fresh orange juice
6 tablespoons fresh lime juice
1 tablespoon peeled and shredded fresh ginger
2 to 3 red chilies, seeded and finely minced
1 teaspoon ground cinnamon
$1/2$ teaspoon ground cardamom
Pinch of ground clove
$1/2$ teaspoon freshly ground black pepper
Sugar, to taste
Salt, to taste
Mint leaves, for garnish

Toss the fruits, coconut, if using, and orange and lime juices in a bowl. In a separate small bowl, combine the ginger, chilies, cinnamon, cardamom, clove, black pepper, sugar, and salt. Gently toss the mixture into the fruit, tossing until all the fruit is coated. Refrigerate, covered, for 2 hours. Serve garnished with mint leaves.

*Yield: 6 to 8 servings*

| | | | |
|---|---|---|---|
| Calories | 127 | Cholesterol | 0 mg |
| Fat | 1 g | Sodium | 22 mg |
| Saturated Fat | 0 g | Carbohydrate | 32 g |
| Mono | 0 g | Protein | 1 g |
| Poly | 0 g | | |

# TROPICAL GRILLED FRUITS WITH LIME YOGURT SAUCE

GRILLING CARAMELIZES the natural sugars of the fruit. The taste of sweet hot fruit right from the grill with a tangy lime yogurt sauce is heavenly.

### Lime Yogurt Sauce
1 cup plain non-fat yogurt
2 teaspoons fresh lime juice
2 teaspoons grated lime zest
Honey, to taste

3 firm bananas, cut in half lengthwise
1 ripe pineapple, peeled, cored, and cut into 1/2-inch slices
2 ripe peaches, peeled and cut into wedges
3 tablespoons brown sugar (optional)
Mint leaves, for garnish

Prepare a charcoal or gas grill. The fire should be medium hot.

Lightly whisk together the yogurt, lime juice, and lime zest in a small bowl. Sweeten with honey. Set aside.

Cut the halved bananas lengthwise into 1/2-inch-thick slices.

Place the fruit on the rack. Grill until the edges of the fruit start to brown, 2 to 3 minutes on each side. If desired, sprinkle brown sugar over the fruit during the last minute of cooking. Remove from the grill. Serve immediately with the lime yogurt sauce.

*Yield: 6 to 8 servings*

| | | | |
|---|---|---|---|
| Calories | 103 | Cholesterol | 1 mg |
| Fat | 1 g | Sodium | 23 mg |
| Saturated Fat | 0 g | Carbohydrate | 25 g |
| Mono | 0 g | Protein | 3 g |
| Poly | 0 g | | |

# CHINESE POACHED PEARS

PEARS POACHED with cinnamon and ginger are the perfect ending to a meal. To the Chinese, pears are the symbol of prosperity.

If the pears are ripe, they may cook in about 5 minutes; if unripe, they may take 30 minutes or longer to become tender.

4 large ripe Bartlett pears, peeled, quartered, and cored
2 tablespoons fresh lemon juice
Grated zest of 1 lemon
$1/3$ cup sugar
2 cinnamon sticks, about 3 inches long
6 slices peeled fresh ginger, about the size of a quarter, smashed

In a bowl, combine the pears, lemon juice, and 1 cup water to prevent them from darkening. Set aside.

In a large pan, combine the grated lemon zest, $3/4$ cup water, sugar, cinnamon sticks, and fresh ginger. Bring to a boil. Reduce the heat and simmer, uncovered, for 5 minutes. Add the pears and soaking liquid. Bring to a simmer. Cover and simmer gently until the pears are tender. Pierce the pears with a sharp knife to determine tenderness. The cooking time depends on the ripeness of the pears. Using a slotted spoon, remove the pears to a serving bowl.

There should be about $1 1/4$ cups of cooking liquid. Bring to a boil and reduce the liquid to about $2/3$ cup. Remove the ginger and cinnamon sticks. Let cool to room temperature. Pour over the cooked pears. Serve.

*Yield: 4 servings*

| | | | |
|---|---|---|---|
| Calories | 165 | Cholesterol | 0 mg |
| Fat | 1 g | Sodium | 0 mg |
| Saturated Fat | 0 g | Carbohydrate | 43 g |
| Mono | 0 g | Protein | 1 g |
| Poly | 0 g | | |

# ORANGE-GLAZED PEARS

AMBER GLAZED pears are a splendid finale to a flavorful Asian meal. Serve the pears alone or with a dollop of lightly beaten non-fat sour cream or yogurt.

   4 ripe Bosc pears with stems intact
   2 tablespoons fresh lemon juice
   1 cup dry white wine
   $1/2$ cup sugar
   2 tablespoons grated orange zest
   2 cinnamon sticks, about 3 inches long
   2 tablespoons orange-flavored liqueur, such as Grand Marnier (optional)
   $1/4$ cup non-fat sour cream or yogurt, lightly beaten (optional)

Preheat the oven to 350 degrees.

   Peel the pears, cut lengthwise in half, and remove the cores. Combine the pears, lemon juice, and water to cover in a bowl, to prevent them from darkening. Set aside.

   Combine the wine, sugar, orange zest, cinnamon sticks, and liqueur, if using, in a saucepan. Bring to a boil, stirring until the sugar is dissolved. Reduce the heat and simmer for 5 minutes.

   Drain the pears. Arrange them on their sides in a baking dish, cut side down. Pour the syrup over the pears. Cover tightly with foil. Bake for about 25 minutes. Turn the pears over and bake for 20 to 30 minutes longer, or until they are tender. Baste 3 times with the syrup during cooking. Remove the foil. Bake the pears for about 10 minutes, basting frequently with the syrup. The pears are done when an amber glaze coats the pears. Be careful not to burn the glaze. Serve the pears warm or allow them to cool and refrigerate, covered. If desired, serve with sour cream or yogurt.

*Yield: 4 servings*

| | | | |
|---|---|---|---|
| Calories | 225 | Cholesterol | 0 mg |
| Fat | 1 g | Sodium | 4 mg |
| Saturated Fat | 0 g | Carbohydrate | 48 g |
| Mono | 0 g | Protein | 1 g |
| Poly | 0 g | | |

# HAUPIA WITH TROPICAL FRUITS

GEORGE MAVROTHALASSITIS, Executive Chef of La Mer Restaurant at the Halekulani Hotel, Honolulu, enhances traditional Hawaiian *haupia* with fresh fruits in season and tops it with a fruit sorbet for a festive dessert.

The haupia can made be made one day in advance, covered with plastic wrap, and refrigerated.

### Haupia
2 envelopes unflavored gelatin
1/2 cup evaporated skim milk
2 tablespoons non-fat dry milk
3 tablespoons plus 2 teaspoons sugar
2 teaspoons almond extract

12 lychees
1 ripe papaya, peeled, seeded, and cut into 1/2-inch cubes
2 ripe mangoes, peeled and cut into 1/2-inch cubes
3 slices ripe pineapple, peeled, cored, and cut into 1/2-inch cubes
1 cantaloupe, seeded and cut into 1/2-inch cubes
1 1/4 cups mango or lime sorbet
4 to 6 sprigs of mint, for garnish

Sprinkle the gelatin over 1/2 cup cold water in a small bowl and let stand until softened, about 1 minute.

Heat, but do not boil, the milk, dry milk, and 3 cups water. Add the sugar and stir to dissolve. Slowly add the softened gelatin and stir over low heat until the gelatin has dissolved completely. Let cool slightly. Stir in the almond extract. Pour into an 8-inch square cake pan. Refrigerate for 4 hours, or until completely set. Cut into 1 1/2-inch diamond shapes.

Combine the fruits in a bowl. Refrigerate for at least 1 hour to allow flavors to marry.

To serve, arrange the fruit and 3 to 4 pieces of the haupia in a soup plate. Place a small scoop of sorbet on top. Garnish with mint leaves.

*Yield: 6 servings*

| | | | |
|---|---|---|---|
| Calories | 238 | Cholesterol | 0 mg |
| Fat | 1 g | Sodium | 83 mg |
| Saturated Fat | 0 g | Carbohydrate | 55 g |
| Mono | 0 g | Protein | 7 g |
| Poly | 0 g | | |

# ALMOND FLOAT WITH RASPBERRY SAUCE

TRADITIONAL CHINESE almond float is served with lots of fresh raspberry sauce.

2 envelopes unflavored gelatin
3$^1/_2$ cups skim milk
2 tablespoons non-fat dry milk
3 tablespoons sugar
1 tablespoon almond extract

*Raspberry Sauce*
1 pound fresh or frozen raspberries
3 tablespoons sugar-free raspberry preserves
1 to 2 tablespoons orange-flavored liqueur, such as Grand Marnier (optional)
8 sprigs of mint

Put an 8- or 9-inch square cake pan in the refrigerator or freezer to chill. Sprinkle the gelatin over $^1/_2$ cup cold water in a small bowl and let stand until softened, about 1 minute.

Combine the milk, dry milk, and sugar in a pan. Bring to a simmer. Stir to dissolve the sugar. Slowly add the softened gelatin and stir over low heat until the gelatin has dissolved. Stir in the almond extract. Pour into the chilled pan. Refrigerate for about 4 hours, or until completely set.

To prepare the sauce, combine 3 cups of the raspberries, the preserves, and $^1/_3$ cup water in a blender or food processor. Puree until smooth. Stir in the orange liqueur, if using. If desired, strain to remove the seeds. Transfer to a bowl or serving container and refrigerate for at least 1 hour.

Cut the chilled almond jelly into 1$^1/_2$-inch diamond-shaped pieces and place on individual serving plates. Pour the chilled raspberry sauce over each portion. Garnish with the remaining raspberries and sprigs of mint.

*Yield: 6 to 8 servings*

| | | | |
|---|---|---|---|
| Calories | 104 | Cholesterol | 2 mg |
| Fat | 1 g | Sodium | 169 mg |
| Saturated Fat | 0 g | Carbohydrate | 20 g |
| Mono | 0 g | Protein | 6 g |
| Poly | 0 g | | |

# JAPANESE LEMON SNOW

## AWAYUKIKAN

HERE IS a light lemony finale served by Motoko Abe, wife of the Consul General of Japan in Chicago. Sliced fresh strawberries or raspberries add a nice touch.

Lemon snow may be prepared a day ahead and refrigerated, covered with plastic wrap.

1 envelope gelatin
1/3 cup plus 2 tablespoons sugar
2 egg whites
1/4 teaspoon cream of tartar
1 teaspoon fresh lemon juice
1/4 teaspoon grated lemon zest
1 tablespoon grated lemon zest, for garnish

Sprinkle the gelatin over 1/4 cup cold water in a small bowl and let stand until softened, about 1 minute.

Dissolve 1/3 cup sugar in 1/2 cup water in a small saucepan over low heat. Add the softened gelatin and stir until just dissolved. Remove from the heat. Add 1/2 cup water. Fill a basin with ice and set the pan in it. Chill until the gelatin mixture has a syrupy consistency. When it begins to set, beat until frothy and more than doubled.

Meanwhile, in the top of a double boiler or a heavy-bottomed saucepan, stir together the egg whites, 1 tablespoon water, the remaining 2 tablespoons of sugar, and cream of tartar. Cook over low heat, beating with a portable mixer at low speed, until the egg whites reach 160 degrees. Scrape the pan, so the whites do not coagulate. Transfer to a large mixing bowl.

Beat the egg whites on high speed until stiff peaks form, about 3 minutes. Stir in lemon juice and 1/4 teaspoon lemon zest and fold the egg whites carefully into the gelatin. Let stand until the mixture begins to thicken. Pour into a wet or lightly oiled 8-inch square cake pan. Refrigerate for 4 hours, or until completely set.

To serve, cut into 1 1/2-inch squares. Serve 2 to 3 pieces to each guest. Sprinkle with lemon zest.

*Yield: 6 to 8 servings*

| Calories | 52 | Cholesterol | 0 mg |
|----------|-----|-------------|------|
| Fat | 0 g | Sodium | 15 mg |
| Saturated Fat | 0 g | Carbohydrate | 12 g |
| Mono | 0 g | Protein | 2 g |
| Poly | 0 g | | |

# SPICED BANANA IN A BANANA LEAF

IN SOUTHEAST Asia and Hawaii, bananas wrapped in banana leaves and grilled or steamed are sold by street vendors as snack foods and as a dessert. The taste varies according to the type of banana. Many exotic bananas can be found today, such as finger-size Mysores with a vanilla-pineapple flavor and black apple-flavored Manzanos. If desired, serve with rum ice cream.

If banana leaves are unavailable, aluminum foil may be substituted. The banana packages may also be steamed for about 20 minutes over boiling water.

1/2 cup honey
1/2 teaspoon ground cinnamon
Banana leaves
4 firm ripe bananas, cut in half
16 mint leaves
2 tablespoons roughly chopped peanuts (optional)

Combine the honey and cinnamon in a bowl.

Pour boiling water over the banana leaves to make them pliable and to prevent splitting. Cut the leaves into eight 12-inch squares.

Place a banana section in the bottom third of the banana leaf. Drizzle the honey and cinnamon mixture over the banana. Place 2 mint leaves on top of each banana piece. Fold into a neat parcel, keeping the seam side on top. Secure with a metal skewer. Grill over medium heat until the bananas are tender but not mushy, 3 to 4 minutes. Serve the bananas in the banana leaf allowing each guest to unwrap his or her own.

*Yield: 6 to 8 servings*

| | | | |
|---|---|---|---|
| Calories | 118 | Cholesterol | 0 mg |
| Fat | 0 g | Sodium | 12 mg |
| Saturated Fat | 0 g | Carbohydrate | 31 g |
| Mono | 0 g | Protein | 1 g |
| Poly | 0 g | | |

# MANGO REFRESHER

THIS VERSION of the favorite hot-weather refresher of India can be varied by using papayas or peaches. If ripe mangoes are unavailable, canned Indian Alphonso mango pulp, available in Indian grocery stores, can be substituted.

2 ripe mangoes, peeled and chopped (about 2 cups)
1½ cups skim milk, chilled
½ cup plain non-fat yogurt
1½ teaspoons vanilla extract
Pinch of salt (optional)
Crushed ice
4 sprigs of mint, for garnish

Using a blender or a handheld immersion blender, whip the mangoes, skim milk, yogurt, vanilla, and salt, if using, together until frothy. Serve immediately over crushed ice. Garnish with mint sprigs.

*Yield: 4 servings*

| | | | |
|---|---|---|---|
| Calories | 121 | Cholesterol | 2 mg |
| Fat | 1 g | Sodium | 71 mg |
| Saturated Fat | 0 g | Carbohydrate | 25 g |
| Mono | 0 g | Protein | 5 g |
| Poly | 0 g | | |

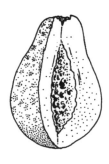

# LEMON GRASS MINT TEA

HERE IS a wonderfully refreshing drink that has rejuvenated me on many a hot day in Thailand. It is important to use only the freshest of lemon grass. For a sweeter tea, add a little honey. Serve over ice.

    12 stalks lemon grass, bottom 6 inches only, smashed with the side of a knife
    1 teaspoon minced mint leaves
    Honey, to taste
    Ice cubes
    4 slices lime

Bring 4 cups of water to a boil. Add the lemon grass and boil for about 15 minutes. Add the mint and honey and stir to dissolve. Let steep for 1 minute. Strain. Refrigerate until chilled. Serve over ice and garnish with lime slices.

*Yield: 4 servings*

| | | | |
|---|---|---|---|
| Calories | 10 | Cholesterol | 0 mg |
| Fat | 0 g | Sodium | 0 mg |
| Saturated Fat | 0 g | Carbohydrate | 0 g |
| Mono | 0 g | Protein | 0 g |
| Poly | 0 g | | |

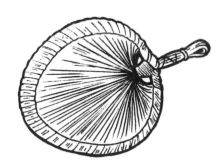

# GINGER TEA

GINGER TEA awakens fond memories of relaxing afternoons in the mountains of Indonesia and of afternoon tea or *merienda* in the Philippines. I often serve the tea after dinner. For a good tea, the ginger must be very fresh.

> 1/3 cup peeled and thinly sliced fresh ginger
> 1/2 cup brown sugar (firmly packed), or to taste

Bring 4 cups of water to a boil. Add the ginger and simmer for 30 minutes, stirring occasionally. Strain. Add the brown sugar and stir to dissolve. Pour into teacups.

*Yield: 4 cups*

| | | | |
|---|---|---|---|
| Calories | 104 | Cholesterol | 0 mg |
| Fat | 0 g | Sodium | 11 mg |
| Saturated Fat | 0 g | Carbohydrate | 27 g |
| Mono | 0 g | Protein | 0 g |
| Poly | 0 g | | |

# MINTED GREEN TEA

A THIRST quencher that is served during the day in Southeast Asia.

3½ cups boiling water
4 teaspoons green tea
8 sprigs of mint, leaves only
6 teaspoons sugar, or to taste

Pour the boiling water into a teapot. Add the green tea and let steep for 3 to 5 minutes. Add the mint leaves and crush with a wooden spoon. Add sugar. Serve hot.

*Yield: 4 servings*

| Calories | 28 | Cholesterol | 0 mg |
|---|---|---|---|
| Fat | 0 g | Sodium | 3 mg |
| Saturated Fat | 0 g | Carbohydrate | 7 g |
| Mono | 0 g | Protein | 0 g |
| Poly | 0 g | | |

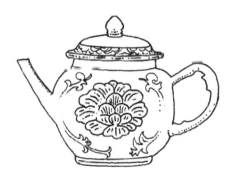

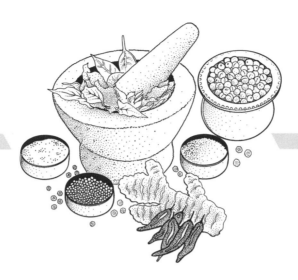

# INGREDIENTS, TECHNIQUES, AND EQUIPMENT

## SPICES, SEASONINGS, AND SPECIAL INGREDIENTS

### ASIAN SESAME OIL (CHINESE SESAME OIL)

An amber-colored, nutty-flavored oil made from toasted white sesame seeds. It is used in small amounts as a flavoring agent. Chinese and Japanese brands are preferable. This oil is totally different from the pressed sesame oil sold in health food stores. There is no substitute.

*Hot sesame oil:* Hot reddish oil made from infusing the heat and flavor of whole dried chilies into sesame oil. It is used as a flavoring to add heat to cooked dishes and as a table condiment.

## Banana leaves

The large, flat green leaves of the banana plant are used to wrap food, to line steamer baskets, to line and decorate elaborate dishes, and as placemats. When used as a wrapper for steamed or grilled food, the leaves impart a delicate, fragrant flavor. They may be purchased frozen in Asian and Hispanic grocery stores. If unavailable, substitute aluminum foil.

## Basil

Holy Basil, Thai Purple Basil, and other Asian basils are often available in Asian grocery stores. Basil is used fresh as an ingredient as well as a garnish. Dried basil cannot be used. European basil can be used.

## Bean curd. *See* tofu.

## Bean sprouts

Mung bean sprouts add texture to many dishes. Purchase crisp sprouts with a fresh smell. If possible, use the sprouts the day of purchase. If not, blanch them in boiling water for 30 seconds, drain, and refresh under cold water. Store in cold water in the refrigerator for 1 day. Do not use canned bean spouts.

## Bean threads. *See* noodles.

## Bonito, dried *(katsuo-bushi)*

Originally, wood-hard wedges of dried bonito, a fish of the mackerel and tuna family, were shaved into flakes over a sharp iron blade. While nothing compares to the flavor of just-shaved bonito, it is a time-consuming process. Today, dried bonito flakes are almost universally used. Dried bonito flakes are sold in small packets in Japanese grocery stores. Open packets should be stored in an airtight container.

## Candlenut *(kemiri)*

A hard, oily nut used for flavoring and as a thickening. Macadamia nuts may be substituted.

## Cardamom

There are two types of cardamom, green and black. Green cardamom is a small half-inch pod that is available in its natural green color or in white form. White cardamom is bleached in the sun and is less aromatic than the green, which has a powerful aroma but a delicate sweet taste. Inside each pod are small brownish-black seeds. Whole pods are slightly crushed and added to delicate rice dishes and desserts to release a warm, aromatic flavor. Often the seeds are removed from the pod, crushed and powdered. I recommend purchasing green cardamom in an Indian grocery store.

*Black cardamom:* Oval pods with a thick dark-brown skin are available only in whole form. The pods are crushed and added to meat and vegetable dishes. Black cardamom is one of the main ingredients in the Indian spice mix known as Garam Masala (page 279). If black cardamom is unavailable, green or white cardamom may be substituted.

CELLOPHANE NOODLES. *See* noodles.

## CHILIES

Chilies, fresh and dried, are used extensively throughout the Pacific Rim. They are a rich source of Vitamins A and C. Since there are many kinds of chilies, and chilies vary in their heat, it might take a little experimentation to determine the number of chilies to use in a dish.

*Fresh chilies:* Choose fresh chilies with skins that are brightly colored and have no brown spots. Though there are exceptions to every rule, especially with regard to chilies, red chilies are generally milder than green chilies. In many Asian dishes, the seeds are not removed, but because most of the heat is in the seeds and veins, they have been removed in recipe directions to leave the rich flavor of the chilies without all of the heat. I have also toned down the heat in the recipes in this book by decreasing the number of chilies. If you want hotter dishes, leave the seeds or increase the number of chilies when cooking. If you wish to add heat to a finished dish, use some red chili sauce.

When handling fresh chilies, you may want to wear rubber gloves. When cutting them, be sure not to touch your eyes or lips and to wash your hands thoroughly with soap and water when finished. Before preparing other foods, wash your knife and chopping block.

*Dried chilies:* These are the sun-dried pods of the capsicum plant. Most of the heat of the dried chilies is concentrated in the seeds. If you wish a milder dish, remove them. They are often soaked in water before being added to a dish.

*Chili bean paste:* In China, chilies are added to fermented soybeans to make this potent paste.

*Chili oil:* Hot reddish oil made from infusing the heat and flavor of whole dried chilies into oil. It is used as a flavoring to add heat to cooked dishes and as a table condiment.

*Chili paste:* This hot seasoning paste is made from ground chilies, garlic, and salt. Different countries have different pastes. In Indonesia and Malaysia, chilies and garlic cooked with vinegar form the base of a bright red paste called sambal ulek. In Korea, a similar sauce, which also includes soybeans, is known as kochujang. A Chinese chili paste with garlic is also imported. Various chili pastes are available in Asian grocery stores.

*Chili sauce:* A hot seasoning sauce prepared from ground chilies and vinegar, differing from country to country. Chinese chili sauce is fairly thick and medium to hot. The Thais like thin, sweet chili sauces, which often look hotter than they are. Vietnamese chili sauces are fiery and intense.

*Red pepper powder:* A powder made from sun-dried or dry-roasted red chili peppers ground to a powder. All recipes in this book have been tested with red pepper powder purchased in Asian grocery stores. Cayenne pepper may be substituted, but chili powder, which is prepared from a combination of ingredients, may not. It will ruin the taste of the dish.

## CHINESE DRIED BLACK MUSHROOMS

Brownish-black dried mushrooms with caps about 1 to 3 inches in diameter impart a distinctive, almost smoky flavor to foods. Large, thick ones with curled edges, light skins, and highly cracked surfaces are the best quality and are generally reserved for banquet dishes and for garnishing. The mushrooms must be soaked in warm water until spongy, 20 to 30 minutes. Stems are rarely used, as they are quite tough. They are available in many supermarkets. Dried shiitakes may be substituted. Dried mushrooms will keep indefinitely if stored in an airtight container.

## CHRYSANTHEMUM LEAVES, EDIBLE *(Shungiku)*

Spicy bright green fragrant leaves often used in Japanese cooking. Available in warm weather.

## CILANTRO. *See* coriander, fresh.

## COCONUT MILK

Coconut milk is used extensively in Southeast Asian and Indian cooking. It has a very high fat content that varies depending upon its thickness. To lower the fat content, yet keep the flavor, I have substituted evaporated skim milk and a small amount of good quality coconut extract or flavoring in some recipes. Wagner's Natural Coconut Flavor is available in gourmet shops and by mail order.

In others, I have used unsweetened ground coconut powder, which can be purchased in Indian grocery stores. If unavailable, grind unsweetened coconut flakes to a powder using a mini processor or blender. Another option is to add Yogurt Cheese (page 280–81) and coconut extract at the end of cooking. This results in a light, slightly tart dish.

## CORIANDER, FRESH (CILANTRO)

Also called Chinese parsley, fresh coriander refers to the leaves of the coriander plant. It has a pungent and agreeable flavor and is used in cooking as well as garnishing. Coriander seeds cannot be used as a substitute.

## CORIANDER SEEDS

Coriander seeds are widely available, both whole and ground, though it is preferable to buy whole seeds and grind them yourself. Toasting brings out the flavor.

## CUMIN SEEDS

These yellow-brown seeds are used whole, crushed, or ground. They are often toasted like sesame seeds (see page 277) to release their rich flavor. It is best to toast and grind your own seeds just before using.

## CURRY LEAVES

Small, shiny, highly aromatic fresh leaves of a tall plant that grows in the Indian subcontinent. They are used in southern Indian and Southeast Asian cooking. When bruised they give a strong fragrance to foods. They are available in Indian grocery stores.

## CURRY POWDER, MADRAS

Western style curry powders are quite different from Indian curry powder and come in many combinations. In India, a combination of spices is blended by the cook. This often varies for each recipe. The best commericial curry powder is from Madras, India. Therefore it is called Madras curry powder.

## DAIKON

A long or large white Asian radish that can grow up to 2 feet in length. It is widely available.

## DASHI (JAPANESE SOUP STOCK). *See* page 61 for recipe.

*Dashi-no-moto (instant Japanese soup stock):* Instant dashi can be dissolved in hot water and used in place of freshly prepared dashi.

## DAUN SALAM

Aromatic Indonesian laurel leaves. Available frozen or dried in Southeast Asian markets. Substitute bay leaf.

## FISH SAUCE

A thin salty, pungent liquid made from fermented fish or shrimp, it is an important seasoning in Southeast Asia. It is milder in flavor than soy sauce. It is called *nam pla* in Thailand, *nuoc mam* in Vietnam, and *patis* in the Philippines.

## FIVE-SPICE POWDER

This Chinese spice powder is a combination of ground star anise, fennel, cinnamon, cloves, and Sichuan peppercorns.

## GALANGAL

Also spelled galingale, this rhizome gives a special aromatic flavor to curries and soups in Southeast Asian dishes. It can be purchased fresh or frozen.

**GARAM MASALA.** *See* page 279 for recipe.

## GINGER

An important ingredient in Asian cooking, this rhizome lends a spicy bite and aroma to dishes. Purchase fresh ginger with a smooth, shiny skin.

> **Pickled ginger:** Thinly sliced pink ginger with a pungent spiciness pickled in sweet vinegar. Available sliced or shredded.

**GYOZA.** *See* potsticker wrappers.

## HOISIN SAUCE

A dark, brownish-red sauce made from fermented beans, salt, sugar, garlic, chilies, sesame seeds, and spices. It is used as a condiment and in marinades for barbecuing and roasting.

## HOT BEAN PASTE

A pungent combination of black beans and chilies, Asian sesame oil, garlic, and sugar. Hot black bean sauce can be substituted.

**HOT SESAME OIL.** *See* Asian sesame oil.

## INDONESIAN SWEET SOY SAUCE *(kecap manis)*

Soy sauce made with a molasses base. It comes bottled in Asian grocery stores.

**JAPANESE HORSERADISH.** *See* wasabi.

## JAPANESE PEPPER POWDER *(sansho)*

The berries of the prickly ash tree called *sansho*. The berries are dried and crushed into powder. The flavor of sansho is tangy rather than hot. Once the package is opened, the sansho should be kept in a tightly sealed container in the refrigerator or freezer.

## JAPANESE SEVEN-SPICE POWDER *(shichimi togarashi)*

Dried red chiles (*togarashi*) are blended with six other herbs and spices (*sansho* pepper, dried tangerine peel, white sesame seeds, dark green *nori*, rape seed and black hemp). There are many blends of the spices. In Japan, they often are mixed to personal taste by local spice blenders. The powder is sold in Japanese markets in small glass jars and should be stored tightly covered in a dark place.

**JAPANESE SWEET RICE WINE.** *See* mirin.

**JAPANESE TARO**

Many types and sizes of taro root exist. Japanese taro is dark skinned, rough textured and about the size of a lemon. Cooked taro is sweet and nutty in flavor. Wear rubber gloves when peeling taro as the juices can be irritating to the skin.

**KAFFIR LIME LEAVES**

The leaves of the kaffir lime tree impart a lemon-lime flavor to many dishes. They are added whole or shredded to curries and soups. The leaves are available fresh, frozen, or dried in Asian grocery stores.

**KECAP MANIS.** *See* Indonesian sweet soy sauce.

**KOCHUJANG.** *See* chili paste.

**KOMBU (DRIED KELP)**
One of the two basic ingredients, the other being bonito flakes, for making the Japanese soup dashi. Many varieties exist. In its natural state, kombu is a deep olive brown from 2½ to 12 inches wide, and several inches to several yards in length.

Kelp has a fine white powder on the surface, which should not be washed off. Before using, lightly wipe with a dampened cloth to remove any foreign matter. Kelp should not boil when making dashi.

When shopping for dried kelp for stock making, ask for *dashi kombu*, kelp for stock making. Generally, the more expensive the kelp, the better the quality and flavor. It is available in Asian markets and so-called wholesome food markets.

**LEMON GRASS**

Stalks of lemon grass are long, hard, and grayish-green. They have a lemony smell. To use fresh lemon grass, peel off the outer layers and use only the bottom 6 inches of the stalk. It may be bruised, sliced crosswise, or ground to a paste (cut thin slices first). Fresh lemon grass can be frozen, well wrapped. If unavailable, the best substitute is very thinly peeled lemon rind, although its taste is not anything like the real thing. When purchasing lemon grass, choose fat, heavy moist stalks.

**MIRIN (JAPANESE SWEET RICE WINE)**

This sweet, syrupy rice wine is an essential Japanese ingredient. It is used in place of sugar to add a mild sweetness to food or to glaze cooked dishes. It is not for drinking purposes. Because its alcohol content is very low, it is sold in grocery not liquor stores.

## Miso

Miso is a salty fermented soybean paste flavored with rice or barley. It is one of Japan's most important staples. Store all miso in the refrigerator for about 6 months. It will lose flavor upon standing.

**White miso (shiro miso):** A sweet and fine-textured miso that is good for light soups and dressings. A favored white miso is *Saikyo miso.*

**Red miso (aka miso):** A combination of barley and soy beans, is saltier than white *miso* and used for hearty soups. *Sendai miso,* named for a northern Japanese city, is considered one of the best red misos.

## Mung beans

Also known as mung dal or green gram. Dried mung beans are sold in Indian grocery stores whole with skins, whole without skin, and split. Fresh mung beans are sprouted for bean sprouts.

## Mushrooms

Mushrooms are used extensively in Asian cuisines. Among the most readily available are Chinese dried black mushrooms (see page 268) and shiitakes.

**Straw mushrooms:** These small light brown mushrooms are crisp, fragrant, and very tasty. They are available in cans in Asian markets and many supermarkets.

## Mustard seeds, black

Tiny black mustard seeds are among the most frequently used spice seeds in South Indian cooking. They are available in Indian grocery stores.

**Nam pla.** *See* fish sauce.

## Noodles

**Bean threads:** Also called cellophane noodles, transparent noodles, glass noodles, these dried, thin, white noodles are made from ground mung beans, and they are sold in small individual packages. They are usually soaked in warm water for 20 minutes before cooking. They are available in Asian grocery stores and most supermarkets.

**Rice sticks:** Also called rice vermicelli or rice flour noodles, these thin, brittle dried noodles made from ground rice need to be rehydrated. For best texture, soak in warm water for 20 minutes before cooking. They should be cooked until tender.

**Soba (Japanese buckwheat noodles):** Thin, brownish gray in color, soba noodles are made from a combination of buckwheat flour, wheat flour, water and salt. They are available fresh and dried.

Dried soba noodles are available at Asian grocery stores and so-called wholesome food stores. For special cooking directions, see page 58.

***Udon noodles (Japanese wheat noodles):*** Wide Japanese white noodles made from wheat and water. Available fresh and dried in Japanese grocery stores and in many supermarkets. They are similar to spaghetti, which can be substituted. Dried noodles will keep indefinitely if stored in an airtight container.

## NORI (SEAWEED)

Nori is the generic term for several seaweeds cultivated in Japan. Nori comes in packages of untoasted or toasted dried sheets. Once the package has been opened, store in an airtight container in a dry, dark place or in the freezer. Toasting nori brings out the flavor and fragrance. To toast, hold a sheet over a gas flame and pass one side over the flame a few times until it becomes crisp.

## NUOC MAM. *See* fish sauce.

## OYSTER-FLAVORED SAUCE

A thick brownish sauce prepared from oyster extracts, sugar, and seasonings. Its rich flavor makes food smooth, subtle and velvety. Store tightly covered in the refrigerator.

## PAPAYA, GREEN

Unripe green papayas are widely used in soups and salads. The small, round black seeds add a peppery taste to salad dressings.

## PLUM SAUCE

An amber sweet-tart sauce made from salted plums, apricots, yams, rice vinegar, chilies, and other spices. It is served as a dipping sauce with roast duck, barbecued meats, and with appetizers. Store covered in refrigerator.

## POTSTICKER WRAPPERS (GYOZA)

Thin, round sheets of pasta dough used to make potstickers. Available in refrigerated section of Asian markets.

## RED PEPPER POWDER. *See* chilies.

## RICE

In Asia and the subcontinent of India, rice is at the forefront of every meal. It is consumed in some form for breakfast, lunch, and dinner. There is short-grain and long-grain rice, including special varieties like basmati rice, grown in India, and jasmine rice, grown in Thailand. Long-grain rice is preferred by most Asians. Short-grain rice is consumed by the Japanese and Koreans. When cooked, short-grain rice is shinier and stickier than long-grain rice. Asians prefer to wash rice before cooking. They feel it gives the rice better texture and taste. Try both ways and decide for yourself.

Nutritional analysis of rice varies from type to type and brand to brand. It can be found on the package.

### Ground Toasted Rice

Put raw long-grain rice in a dry skillet over medium heat. Toast, stirring frequently, until the rice is light golden brown, 4 to 5 minutes. Remove from the heat. Let the rice cool to room temperature. In a mortar, mini processor, blender, or coffee grinder, pound or grind the rice to a coarse powder. Toasted rice will keep for 6 months in an airtight container.

*Long-grain rice:* Long-grain rice cooks up dry and fluffy and has grains that separate easily. The amount of water used when cooking rice will vary upon the strain and age of the rice and the depth of the pan. Therefore, the measurements given are approximate.

### Steamed Long-grain Rice

1 cup long-grain rice
$1^3/_4$ to 2 cups water

Place the rice in a container and add water to cover by at least 1 inch. Rub the grains together between the palms of your hands until the water becomes cloudy. Pour the rice into a colander to drain. Repeat the washing 3 to 5 times, or until the water is clear. Drain thoroughly.

Place the rice in a heavy 2-quart saucepan that has a tight-fitting lid. Bring to a boil, uncovered, over high heat. Reduce the heat, cover the pan, and simmer until all the water is absorbed, 15 to 20 minutes. Do not lift the cover during this time. Toward the end of this period, open the cover only long enough to check to see that all the water has been absorbed. Cover again. Turn off the heat and let stand for 10 minutes. Fluff the rice with a fork. Serve warm.

*Yield: 3 cups*

*Basmati rice:* Aromatic long-grain basmati rice has a distinctive nutty flavor and grows in the foothills of the Himalayas. The best basmati can be purchased in Indian, Pakistani, and Persian grocery stores. The amount of water for cooking the rice will depend upon the age and strain of rice. Therefore the amounts given are approximate. For best results, soak the rice before cooking.

### Steamed Basmati Rice

1 cup basmati rice
$1^2/_3$ to 2 cups water

Spread out the rice on a flat surface. Pick it over and discard all foreign matter. Put the rice in a container and rub the grains together between the palms of your hands until the water becomes cloudy. Pour the rice into a strainer to drain. Repeat the washing procedure 3 to 5 times, or until the water is clear. Drain thoroughly. Put the rice in a bowl. Add water to cover the rice by at least 1 inch. Soak the rice for at least 20 minutes to allow the grains to expand. Drain the rice, reserving the soaking water.

Bring 1²/₃ to 2 cups of the soaking water to a boil in a heavy-bottomed 2-quart saucepan. Add the drained rice and stir carefully. Bring the rice to a boil, stirring gently. Reduce the heat to low and simmer, partially covered, until most of the water is absorbed and the surface of the rice is full of craters, 10 to 15 minutes. Cover the pan with a tight lid. If you do not have a tight lid, cover the pan with aluminum foil and place the lid on top of the foil to produce a tight seal. Reduce the heat to the lowest setting and raise the pan 1 inch above the burner. (This can be done on a heat diffuser or wok ring.) Steam the rice for about 10 minutes. Let the rice rest, covered, for about 5 minutes. Fluff the rice with a fork. Cooked rice will remain warm for about 20 minutes. Serve.

*Yield: about 3 cups*

**Short-grain rice:** Short-grain rice is popular in Japan and Korea. When cooked, it is shiny and sticky in texture. The amount of water needed for cooking varies depending on the strain and age of the rice and the size of the pan. Use the smaller amount if you want firm rice, the greater if you want soft rice. Newly harvested rice that comes to market in October would have only enough water to equal the amount of dry rice.

### Steamed Short-grain Rice

1 cup short-grain rice
1¹/₈ to 1¹/₄ cups water

Put the rice in a container. Add water to cover by at least 1 inch and rub the grains together between the palms of your hands until the water becomes cloudy. Pour the rice into a colander to drain. Repeat the washing procedure 3 to 5 times, or until the water is almost clear. Rinse the rice thoroughly with water. Drain. Put the rice in a heavy 1 quart saucepan that has a tight-fitting lid. Pour the water over the rice. Let the rice soak for 30 minutes.

Cook the rice, tightly covered, over medium heat until the water just boils. Turn the heat to high and let the water and the cover bounce up and down, about 4 to 5 minutes. A white, starchy liquid will bubble from under the cover. When this bubbling stops, reduce the heat to medium-low and continue cooking for about 8 to 10 minutes, or until all the water has been absorbed. Do not lift the cover during cooking. Turn off the heat and let the cooked rice steam for 15 to 20 minutes. Fluff with a wooden paddle or spoon. Serve. If not serving immediately, place a towel between the cover and the pan to absorb the moisture before serving.

*Yield: about 2 cups*

**Glutinous rice:** Very white, short-grained rice. The starchiest of all rices, it has a sweet, sticky consistency when cooked.

**Steamed Glutinous Rice**

1 cup glutinous rice
1½ cups water

Put the rice in a large bowl with water to cover by about 2 inches. Swish the water around with your fingers to remove the starch coating on the grains. Drain the rice and continue this process until the water is no longer milky. Drain.

Line a covered steamer basket with moistened cheesecloth. Spread the rice in the basket in an even layer. Steam over boiling water for 25 minutes, or until soft. Serve hot, warm, or at room temperature.

*Yield: about 1¾ cups*

*Sushi rice: See* Vinegared Rice for Sushi (page 44).

### How to Cook Rice in an Automatic Rice Cooker

Measure the rice and water and wash and soak as described on page 274. Put the rice and water into the cooker. Start the cooker about 25 minutes before desired serving time. The actual cooking time is about 10 to 15 minutes. The cooker bell will go off, but do not remove the cover. Steaming will take another 10 to 15 minutes. When the steaming is completed, remove the cover and fluff the rice with a wooden paddle. The rice is ready to serve. If not serving immediately, place a towel between the cover and the pan to absorb the moisture before serving. One cup of rice cooks up to about 2½ cups of cooked rice.

## RICE PAPER WRAPPERS

Round tissue-thin sheets of "paper" made of rice, salt, and water. They are available in 6½-, 8½-, and 13½-inch sizes in Asian markets.

## RICE STICKS (RICE VERMICELLI). *See* noodles.

## SAFFRON THREADS

The world's most expensive spice, saffron is the dried stigmas of the saffron crocus. The dark orange, threadlike strands give food a yellow color and a distinctive aroma and taste. Always purchase saffron threads, not powder.

## SAKE (JAPANESE RICE WINE)

Sake is consumed as a beverage and is an important ingredient in Japanese cooking. Its basic ingredients are rice, a fermenting agent, and water.

## SAMBAL ULEK. *See* chili sauce.

**SANSHO.** *See* Japanese pepper powder.

**SESAME OIL.** *See* Asian sesame oil.

## SESAME SEEDS

Both white and black sesame seeds are used to flavor and garnish dishes. White sesame seeds have a sweet, nutty flavor and should be toasted before using. Black sesame seeds are slightly bitter.

### *How to Toast Sesame Seeds*

Toast the sesame seeds in a dry skillet over medium-high heat for 30 seconds, or until they are light brown. Shake the pan to prevent them from burning. Remove from the pan immediately. Let cool. Place in a mortar or shallow bowl. Pound the sesame seeds with a pestle or a blunt rounded object such as a wooden spoon handle, grinding them until flaky. The toasted seeds may also be placed in a heavy-duty plastic bag and crushed with a rolling pin.

## SHALLOTS

Small, purplish onions with red-brown skin. Roasted shallots are used as a garnish for soups, salads, and stir-fries in many Southeast Asian and Indian dishes. The shallots are usually deep-fried; oven-roasting provides a healthful alternative. If shallots are unavailable, substitute a smaller amount of yellow onion.

### Crisp Roasted Shallots

Vegetable oil spray
6 large shallots, thinly sliced
Salt, to taste (optional)

Preheat the oven to 400 degrees. Spray a nonstick baking sheet lightly with oil. Sprinkle the shallot slices over the baking sheet. Spray oil evenly over the shallots. Bake in the center of the oven, stirring occasionally, for about 15 minutes, or until brown and crisp. If desired, season lightly with salt. Let cool completely. Store in an airtight container in the refrigerator for up to 10 days.

*Yield: about ¹/₃ cup*

**SHICHIMI TOGARASHI.** *See* Japanese seven-spice powder.

## SHRIMP, DRIED

Bright orange tiny dried shrimps have a unique flavor. They are used in soups, stir-fries, noodles, vegetables, and salads. Sold in small packs. Store in an airtight container.

## SICHUAN (SZECHWAN) PEPPERCORNS

Reddish-brown, open-husked peppercorns (actually the berries of the prickly ash tree rather than true peppercorns) with a strong flavor. They are often dry-roasted to bring out their flavor and fragrance.

## SICHUAN (SZECHWAN) PRESERVED MUSTARD GREENS

Spicy-salty tasting preserved mustard greens are pickled in vinegar with salt and chili powder. To reduce the saltiness, rinse with water to remove excess pickling brine. Available in cans.

## SOBA. *See* noodles.

## SOY SAUCE

This important ingredient in Asian cooking is prepared from fermented soybeans and wheat, using a natural fermentation process.

*Soy sauce, reduced sodium:* About 40 percent less sodium than regular soy sauce. Because it has less sodium than regular soy sauce, it must be refrigerated after opening.

## SPICES

Spices play an important role in high-flavor cooking. It is best to purchase spices whole and grind them as needed. If you find this impractical, store ground spices in an airtight container in a cool, dark, dry place for 3 to 4 months. Whole spices will keep up to 1 year. Freezing whole spices keeps them fresh longer.

### How to Roast Spices

Heat a heavy pan over medium heat. Add the spice and roast, shaking and stirring the pan constantly. Be careful not to let the spice burn. When it starts to brown, remove the spice from the pan immediately. Let cool.

### How to Grind Spices

Grind small amounts of spice to a fine powder in a mortar, spice mill, or coffee grinder reserved for spices. If you do not have a grinder, place the spice on wax paper. Cover with another layer of wax paper and roll with a rolling pin or pound with a kitchen mallet or the flat bottom of a kitchen pan. Ground spices may be stored in an airtight container for 3 months.

## SPICE MIXTURES

Spice mixtures increase the intensity of foods and play an important role in low-fat cooking. A mortar and pestle can handle small quantities, mashing the ingredients into a smooth paste and releasing flavors more effectively than a machine. To save time, small amounts of paste mixtures can be processed in a mini processor or in a blender. When preparing a paste mixture, chop the large and hard ingredients by hand, then add them to the mortar, mini processor or blender. If necessary, add a little liquid to produce a smooth paste.

Dry spice blends also add aroma and flavor to dishes. Garam Masala is an Indian blend of dry-roasted spices. It is best when freshly made.

### Garam Masala

2 tablespoons black cardamom pods
1 stick cinnamon, 2 inches, crushed
2 teaspoons whole cloves
4 teaspoons black peppercorns

Roast the spices separately in a dry skillet over medium heat, stirring until aromatic. Be careful not to let the spices burn. In a mortar, spice mill, clean electric coffee grinder, or mini processor, pound or grind to a fine powder. Store in an airtight container away from heat and light for 2 to 3 months.

*Yield: about 6 tablespoons*

| Calories | 14 | Carbohydrate | 3 g |
|----------|-----|--------------|------|
| Sodium | 1 mg | Cholesterol | 0 mg |
| Fat | 0 g | Protein | 1 g |

## STAR ANISE

A dried star-shape spice. It has a licorice flavor and is used as a seasoning in marinades, braised dishes, and stews.

## TAMARIND

The beanlike pod of the tamarind tree contains seeds and a pulp that has a tart citrus flavor. Prepared pulp is sold in Asian markets. Some Thai and Indian grocery stores sell a concentrate that can be diluted with water before use. When the amount of tamarind needed is small, I use the concentrate. When larger amount is needed, I prefer to use tamarind puree, which has a richer taste and flavor.

### Tamarind Liquid

1 teaspoon tamarind pulp
2 teaspoons hot water

Combine the tamarind and hot water in a small bowl. Let soak for 20 to 30 minutes, squeezing the pulp with your fingers to break it apart and separate the strings. Strain the liquid through a fine sieve, forcing the pulp against the strainer. Reserve the liquid and discard the pulp. Use immediately or store in a tightly covered glass container in the refrigerator for 2 to 3 days.

**TARO, JAPANESE.** *See* Japanese taro.

## TOFU

Called bean curd in most of Asia, but marketed as tofu (its Japanese name) in the United States. There are three basic types: firm, regular, and soft. Widely available in plastic containers in refrigerated section of most supermarkets. It will keep refrigerated for several days if water is changed daily.

*Firm tofu:* Used for stir-fried dishes, stews, and other dishes in which the bean curd should retain its shape.

*Regular tofu:* Can be crumbled and tossed into salads.

*Soft tofu:* Has a custard-like consistency and is used in soups and salad dressings.

## TURMERIC

A yellow-orange rhizome similar to ginger in appearance, it grows underground in Southeast Asia and India. Turmeric imparts a pleasingly pungent flavor to dishes. Fresh turmeric root is rarely seen in the United States. In Asia, fresh turmeric is boiled and sun-dried, then ground to a powder. It is available here in this form.

**UDON NOODLES.** *See* noodles.

## WASABI (JAPANESE HORSERADISH)

A fiery condiment used for sashimi and sushi. Wasabi comes powdered in small round tins or as a ready-to-use paste in small tubes. To prepare the powdered wasabi, add a small amount of warm water to a small amount of the powder. Stir until smooth. Let the paste mixture stand, covered, for 15 minutes to allow the flavors to develop. Wasabi loses it heat with exposure to air. Prepare only as much as you will use at a sitting.

## WONTON WRAPPERS

Made from wheat flour, water, and eggs, these 3½-inch squares hold a variety of dumpling fillings. Store in refrigerator for up to 1 week.

## YOGURT CHEESE

Yogurt cheese is made by draining yogurt in a fine-meshed strainer. Yogurt cheese made with non-fat yogurt can be used in spreads and dips or as a base for sauces. The longer you drain the yogurt, the firmer the cheese will be.

**Yogurt Cheese**

1 quart plain non-fat yogurt

Put the yogurt in a fine-mesh strainer over a bowl. If you do not have a fine-mesh strainer, line a strainer with a coffee filter or several layers of cheesecloth and use that. Cover and let drain in the refrigerator for 5 hours or overnight.

*Yield: 2 cups*

| | | | |
|---|---|---|---|
| Calories | 60 | Cholesterol | 3 mg |
| Fat | 0 g | Sodium | 80 mg |
| Saturated Fat | 0 g | Carbohydrate | 9 g |
| Mono | 0 g | Protein | 7 g |
| Poly | 0 g | | |

# SPECIAL TECHNIQUES

In the high heat and faster cooking in stir-frying, the food must be cut uniformly in order for it to cook evenly. The first thing the eye sees is the color, size, and shape of a dish. To Asians, each ingredient should be cut as specified in a recipe because the size and shape of the cut ingredients are as important as the taste.

## CUTTING TECHNIQUES

*Julienne cutting:* Cut the food into slices of desired length, usually about 1½ to 2 inches. Stack the slices and slice down through the stack into matchstick sticks, which are square in cross section.

*Dicing:* Cut the food into slices. Stack the slices on top of each other and cut them lengthwise into strips. Stack the strips and cut crosswise into evenly sized cubes or dice. (When making a paste mixture, it is not necessary to chop the food evenly. You may roughly chop it.)

*Mincing:* To mince an ingredient is to cut it into very small pieces, about 1/16 inch.

*Smashing, crushing, and bruising:* Ginger, garlic, lemon grass, and other ingredients are often crushed to release their flavors. Cut to the desired size. Place the pieces on a cutting board and hit firmly with the flat side of a knife blade. This can also be done before mincing an ingredient, making the process easier.

## COOKING TECHNIQUES

*Stir-frying and sautéing:* Stir-frying is one of the most basic cooking techniques of the Pacific Rim. A nonstick stir-fry pan or wok is ideal for stir-frying, but you may also use a large nonstick skillet.

High-quality nonstick pans are essential for light cooking. The pans used for both stir-frying and sautéing should be large enough that the food is not crowded. If the food does not fit easily, the cooking should be done in batches. If you overload the pan, you will braise the food and the ingredients will not be crisp.

Because stir-frying is extremely fast, organization of the foods before cooking is of utmost importance. Organize all of the ingredients, utensils, and equipment before starting to cook. Heat the nonstick pan over moderately high heat. Add a little oil or lightly spray the pan if necessary. Add each ingredient as specified and cook to the desired doneness. Ingredients requiring different cooking times are often added separately. Add the specified amount of ingredients in each recipe. If doubling a recipe or cooking more food than called for, cook the food in batches.

Sautéing means to cook food briefly in a little oil over medium-high heat.

**Steaming:** Steaming is very important in cooking in a healthy manner. It is a nutritious method of preparing food, since vitamins and minerals are preserved, rather than being diminished by boiling. It is also important in light cooking because no fat is used.

When steaming, the food should be suspended at least $1\frac{1}{2}$ to 2 inches above the surface of the boiling water so that no water touches the cooking food and the steam circulates properly. The water in the steamer must be boiling before the food is placed in the container. Check the water level occasionally to be sure that it has not boiled away. When checking the food to see if it is done, carefully remove the lid, holding it away from you in order to avoid the steam. Chinese bamboo steamers or metal steaming pots with several steaming inserts allow several layers of food to be steamed at once.

**Blanching:** Vegetables are frequently plunged into a large pan of boiling water and cooked rapidly to keep them crisp and their color bright. Cook until almost tender but still crunchy, drain immediately, then rinse under cold running water to stop the cooking process.

## SPECIAL EQUIPMENT

The only thing essential is good quality nonstick pans. Flat-bottomed nonstick stir-fry pans are especially useful.

INGREDIENTS CAN BE PURCHASED IN ASIAN MARKETS,
SOME SPECIALTY FOOD SHOPS,
AND IN MOST CASES BY MAIL ORDER FROM:

Adriana's Caravan
409 Vanderbilt Street
New York, NY 11218
(800) 316-0820

Balducci's
Shop from Home Service
42–26 13th Street
Long Island City, NY 11101
(800) 225-3822

Dean & DeLuca
560 Broadway
New York, NY 10012
(800) 221-7714

Foods of India
120 Lexington Avenue
New York, NY 10016
(212) 683-4419

Kalustyan's
123 Lexington Avenue
New York, NY 10016
(212) 685-3451

Katagiri
224 East 59th Street
New York, NY 10022
(212) 755-3566

Penzey's Spice House
P.O. Box 1448
Waukesha, WI 53187
(414) 579-0277

Spice Merchant
P.O. Box 524
Jackson Hole, WY 83001
(800) 551-5999

Zabar's
Mail Order Department
2245 Broadway
New York, NY 10024
(800) 697-6301

# BIBLIOGRAPHY

Aziz, Khalid; Hsiung, Deh-Ta; Kazuko, Emi; Morris, Sallie. *Oriental Gourmet*. New York: Gallery Books, 1986

Andoh, Elizabeth. *An American Taste of Japan*. New York: William Morrow and Company, 1985.

_____. *At Home with Japanese Cooking*. New York: Alfred A. Knopf, 1980.

Brackman, Agnes de Keijzer. *Art of Indonesian Cooking*. Singapore: Asia Pacific Press, 1970.

Brennan, Jennifer. *The Cuisines of Asia*. New York: St. Martin's Press, 1984.

Brissenden, Rosemary. *Southeast Asian Food (Indonesia, Malaysia and Thailand)*. Middlesex, England: Penguin Books, 1969.

Burum, Linda. *Asian Pasta: A Cook's Guide to the Noodles, Wrappers and Pasta Creations of the East*. Berkeley: Aris Books, 1985.

*Chefs in Paradise*. Honolulu: Hawaii Stars Presents, Inc., 1994.

Claiborne, Craig, and Lee, Virginia. *The Chinese Cookbook*. Philadelphia and New York: J. B. Lippincott Company, 1972.

Dal, Tarla. *Indian Vegetarian Cooking*. London: Ebury Press, 1986.

Devi, Yamuna. *Lord Krishna's Cuisine: The Art of Indian Vegetarian Cooking*. New York: E. P. Dutton/ Bala Books, 1987.

Han, Chung Hea. *For Your Health Korean Cooking*. Seoul: Chung Woo Publishing Co., 1985.

Harris, Marilyn Rittenhouse. *Tropical Fruit Cookbook*. Honolulu: University of Hawaii Press, 1993.

Hom, Ken. *Ken Hom's Chinese Cookery*. New York: Harper & Row, 1986.

Jeong, Ha Sook. *Traditional Korean Cooking*. Seoul: Soodo Publishing Co., 1985.

Kalra, J. Inder Singh, and Gupta, Pradeep Dar. *Prashad: Cooking with the Indian Masters*. New Delhi: Allied Publishers, Ltd., 1990.

Law, Ruth. *Dim Sum: Fast and Festive Chinese Cooking*. Chicago: Contemporary Books, 1982.

_____. *The Southeast Asia Cookbook*. New York: Donald I. Fine, Inc., 1990.

_____. *Indian Light Cooking*. New York: Donald I. Fine, Inc., 1994.

Lee, Mrs. Chin Koon. *Mrs. Lee's Cookbook*. Singapore: Lee Chin Koon, 1974.

Ortiz, Elizabeth Lambert, with Endo, Mitsuko. *The Complete Book of Japanese Cooking*. New York: Gallahad Books, 1994.

Owen, Sri. *Indonesian Food and Cookery*. London: Prospect Books, 1986.

Peterson, James. *Fish & Shellfish*. New York: William Morrow and Company, 1996.

Rombauer, Irma, and Rombauer, Marion Becker. *Joy of Cooking*. New York: Scribner's, 1995.

Sakai, Miyoko, and Abe, Motoko. *Quick & Easy Japanese Cooking for Everyone.* Tokyo: The Japan Times, 1989.

Sahni, Julie. *Classic Indian Cooking.* New York: William Morrow and Company, 1980.

Schlesinger, Chris, and Willoughby, John. *The Thrill of the Grill.* New York: William Morrow and Company, 1990.

Schlesinger, Chris, and Willoughby, John. *Salsas, Sambals, Chutneys & Chowchows.* New York: William Morrow and Company, 1993.

Scott, David. *Indonesian Cookery.* London: Rider and Company, 1984.

Shenoy, Jaya. *Dakshin Bharat Cookbook.* Manipal, India: Manipal Power Press, 1989.

Simonds, Nina. *Classic Chinese Cuisine.* Boston: Houghton Mifflin Company, 1982.

Solomon, Charmaine. *The Complete Asian Cookbook.* Sydney: Weldons, 1990.

Steinberg, Rafail. *The Cooking of Japan.* New York: Time-Life Books, 1969.

Stuart, Ann Thu. *Vietnamese Cooking.* Sydney: Angus and Robertson, 1986.

Tropp, Barbara. *The Modern Art of Chinese Cooking.* New York: William Morrow and Company, 1982.

Tsuji, Shizuo. *Japanese Cooking: A Simple Art.* Toyko: Kodansha International, 1980.

Takahashi, Kuwaka. *The Joy of Japanese Cooking.* Tokyo: Shufunotomo Co., Ltd., 1986.

Wade, Lee. *Lee Wade's Korean Cookery.* Seoul: Hollym Corporation, 1985.

Yan, Martin. *Culinary Journey Through China.* San Francisco: KQED Books, 1995.

## U.S. AND METRIC CONVERSION TABLE

| Symbol | When you know | Multiply by | To find |
|---|---|---|---|
| **VOLUME** | | | |
| tsp | teaspoons | 5.0 | milliliters |
| tbsp | tablespoons | 15.0 | milliliters |
| fl oz. | fluid ounces | 29.57 | milliliters |
| c | cups | 0.24 | liters |
| pt | pints | 0.47 | liters |
| qt | quarts | 0.95 | liters |
| gal | gallons | 3.8 | liters |
| ml | milliliters | 0.034 | fluid ounces |
| **MASS (Weight)** | | | |
| oz | ounces | 28.35 | grams |
| lb | pounds | 0.45 | kilograms |
| g | grams | 0.035 | ounces |
| kg | kilograms | 2.2 | pounds |
| **TEMPERATURE** | | | |
| °F | Farenheit | 5/9 (after subtracting 32) | Celsius |
| **LENGTH** | | | |
| in | inches | 2.5 | centimeters |

## QUICK ROUNDED MEASUREMENTS FOR EASY REFERENCE

| VOLUME | | | | | | MASS (Weight) | | |
|---|---|---|---|---|---|---|---|---|
| 1/4 tsp | = | 1/24 oz | = | 1 ml | | 1 oz | = | 30 g |
| 1/2 tsp | = | 1/12 oz | = | 2 ml | | 4 oz | = | 115 g |
| 1 tsp | = | 1/6 oz | = | 5 ml | | 8 oz | = | 225 g |
| 1 tbsp | = | 1/2 oz | = | 15 ml | | 16 oz (1 lb) | = | 450 g |
| 1 c | = | 8 oz | = | 250 ml | | 32 oz (2 lb) | = | 900 g |
| 4 c (1 qt) | = | 32 oz | = | 1 liter | | 36 oz (2 1/4 lb) | = | 1000 g (1kg) |

# INDEX

3199 7x
8/03 LAD 03/01 15x